BLACKWELL'S
UNDERGROUND CLINICAL VIGNETTES

PATHOPHYSIOLOGY
VOL. III, 3E

BLACKWELL'S
UNDERGROUND CLINICAL VIGNETTES

PATHOPHYSIOLOGY VOL. III, 3E

VIKAS BHUSHAN, MD
University of California, San Francisco, Class of 1991
Series Editor, Diagnostic Radiologist

VISHAL PALL, MBBS
Government Medical College, Chandigarh, India, Class of 1996
Series Editor, U. of Texas, Galveston, Resident in Internal Medicine &
Preventive Medicine

TAO LE, MD
University of California, San Francisco, Class of 1996

ASHRAF ZAMAN, MBBS
New Delhi, India

Blackwell
Science

CONTRIBUTORS

Robert Nason
University of Texas Medical Branch, Class of 2003

Kristen Lem Mygdal, MD
University of Kansas School of Medicine, Resident in Radiology

Kalpita Shah, PA-C
University of Texas Medical Branch, Galveston, Class of 2000

Fadi Abu Shahin, MD
University of Damascus, Syria, Class of 1999

Hoang Nguyen, MD, MBA
Northwestern University, Class of 2001

Sonal Shah, MD
Ross University, Class of 2000

© 2002 by Blackwell Science, Inc.

Editorial Offices:
Commerce Place, 350 Main Street, Malden,
    Massachusetts 02148, USA
Osney Mead, Oxford OX2 0EL, England
25 John Street, London WC1N 2BS, England
23 Ainslie Place, Edinburgh EH3 6AJ, Scotland
54 University Street, Carlton, Victoria 3053,
    Australia

Other Editorial Offices:
Blackwell Wissenschafts-Verlag GmbH,
    Kurfürstendamm 57, 10707 Berlin, Germany
Blackwell Science KK, MG Kodenmacho Building,
    7–10 Kodenmacho Nihombashi, Chuo-ku,
    Tokyo 104, Japan
Iowa State University Press, A Blackwell Science
    Company, 2121 S. State Avenue, Ames, Iowa
    50014-8300, USA

Acquisitions: Laura DeYoung
Development: Amy Nuttbrock
Production: Lorna Hind and Shawn Girsberger
Manufacturing: Lisa Flanagan
Marketing Manager: Kathleen Mulcahy
Cover design by Leslie Haimes
Interior design by Shawn Girsberger
Typeset by TechBooks
Printed and bound by Capital City Press

Blackwell's Underground Clinical Vignettes:
    Pathophysiology III, 3e
ISBN 0-632-04555-8

Printed in the United States of America
02 03 04 05 5 4 3 2 1

First Indian Reprint 2002

Printed and bound by Multivista Global Limited,
Chennai - 600 042.

The Blackwell Science logo is a trade mark of
Blackwell Science Ltd., registered at the United
Kingdom Trade Marks Registry

Library of Congress Cataloging-in-Publication Data
Bhushan, Vikas.
Blackwell's underground clinical vignettes.
Pathophysiology / author, Vikas Bhushan. – 3rd ed.
    p. ; cm. – (Underground clinical vignettes)
Rev. ed. of: Pathophysiology / Vikas Bhushan. 2nd ed.
c1999. ISBN 0-632-04551-5 (pbk.)
1. Physiology, Pathological – Case studies.
2. Physicians – Licenses – United States –
Examinations – Study guides.
    [DNLM: 1. Clinical Medicine – Case Report.
2. Clinical Medicine – Problems and Exercises.
WB 18.2 B575bb 2002] I. Title: Underground
clinical vignettes. Pathophysiology. II. Pathophysiology.
III. Title. IV. Series.
    RB113 .B459 2002
    616.07'076–dc21

                                                2001004931

Notice

The authors of this volume have taken care that the information contained herein is accurate and compatible with the standards generally accepted at the time of publication. Nevertheless, it is difficult to ensure that all the information given is entirely accurate for all circumstances. The publisher and authors do not guarantee the contents of this book and disclaim any liability, loss, or damage incurred as a consequence, directly or indirectly, of the use and application of any of the contents of this volume.

CONTENTS

ACKNOWLEDGMENTS

Throughout the production of this book, we have had the support of many friends and colleagues. Special thanks to our support team including Anu Gupta, Andrea Fellows, Anastasia Anderson, Srishti Gupta, Mona Pall, Jonathan Kirsch and Chirag Amin. For prior contributions we thank Gianni Le Nguyen, Tarun Mathur, Alex Grimm, Sonia Santos and Elizabeth Sanders.

We have enjoyed working with a world-class international publishing group at Blackwell Science, including Laura DeYoung, Amy Nuttbrock, Lisa Flanagan, Shawn Girsberger, Lorna Hind and Gordon Tibbitts. For help with securing images for the entire series we also thank Lee Martin, Kristopher Jones, Tina Panizzi and Peter Anderson at the University of Alabama, the Armed Forces Institute of Pathology, and many of our fellow Blackwell Science authors.

For submitting comments, corrections, editing, proofreading, and assistance across all of the vignette titles in all editions, we collectively thank:

Tara Adamovich, Carolyn Alexander, Kris Alden, Henry E. Aryan, Lynman Bacolor, Natalie Barteneva, Dean Bartholomew, Debashish Behera, Sumit Bhatia, Sanjay Bindra, Dave Brinton, Julianne Brown, Alexander Brownie, Tamara Callahan, David Canes, Bryan Casey, Aaron Caughey, Hebert Chen, Jonathan Cheng, Arnold Cheung, Arnold Chin, Simion Chiosea, Yoon Cho, Samuel Chung, Gretchen Conant, Vladimir Coric, Christopher Cosgrove, Ronald Cowan, Karekin R. Cunningham, A. Sean Dailey, Rama Dandamudi, Sunit Das, Ryan Armando Dave, John David, Emmanuel de la Cruz, Robert DeMello, Navneet Dhillon, Sharmila Dissanaike, David Donson, Adolf Etchegaray, Alea Eusebio, Priscilla A. Frase, David Frenz, Kristin Gaumer, Yohannes Gebreegziabher, Anil Gehi, Tony George, L.M. Gotanco, Parul Goyal, Alex Grimm, Rajeev Gupta, Ahmad Halim, Sue Hall, David Hasselbacher, Tamra Heimert, Michelle Higley, Dan Hoit, Eric Jackson, Tim Jackson, Sundar Jayaraman, Pei-Ni Jone, Aarchan Joshi, Rajni K. Jutla, Faiyaz Kapadi, Seth Karp, Aaron S. Kesselheim, Sana Khan, Andrew Pin-wei Ko, Francis Kong, Paul Konitzky, Warren S. Krackov, Benjamin H.S. Lau, Ann LaCasce, Connie Lee, Scott Lee, Guillermo Lehmann, Kevin Leung, Paul Levett, Warren Levinson, Eric Ley, Ken Lin,

Pavel Lobanov, J. Mark Maddox, Aram Mardian, Samir Mehta, Gil Melmed, Joe Messina, Robert Mosca, Michael Murphy, Vivek Nandkarni, Siva Naraynan, Carvell Nguyen, Linh Nguyen, Deanna Nobleza, Craig Nodurft, George Noumi, Darin T. Okuda, Adam L. Palance, Paul Pamphrus, Jinha Park, Sonny Patel, Ricardo Pietrobon, Riva L. Rahl, Aashita Randeria, Rachan Reddy, Beatriu Reig, Marilou Reyes, Jeremy Richmon, Tai Roe, Rick Roller, Rajiv Roy, Diego Ruiz, Anthony Russell, Sanjay Sahgal, Urmimala Sarkar, John Schilling, Isabell Schmitt, Daren Schuhmacher, Sonal Shah, Fadi Abu Shahin, Mae Sheikh-Ali, Edie Shen, Justin Smith, John Stulak, Lillian Su, Julie Sundaram, Rita Suri, Seth Sweetser, Antonio Talayero, Merita Tan, Mark Tanaka, Eric Taylor, Jess Thompson, Indi Trehan, Raymond Turner, Okafo Uchenna, Eric Uyguanco, Richa Varma, John Wages, Alan Wang, Eunice Wang, Andy Weiss, Amy Williams, Brian Yang, Hany Zaky, Ashraf Zaman and David Zipf.

For generously contributing images to the entire *Underground Clinical Vignette* Step 1 series, we collectively thank the staff at Blackwell Science in Oxford, Boston, and Berlin as well as:

- Axford, J. *Medicine.* Osney Mead: Blackwell Science Ltd, 1996. Figures 2.14, 2.15, 2.16, 2.27, 2.28, 2.31, 2.35, 2.36, 2.38, 2.43, 2.65a, 2.65b, 2.65c, 2.103b, 2.105b, 3.20b, 3.21, 8.27, 8.27b, 8.77b, 8.77c, 10.81b, 10.96a, 12.28a, 14.6, 14.16, 14.50.

- Bannister B, Begg N, Gillespie S. *Infectious Disease, 2nd Edition.* Osney Mead: Blackwell Science Ltd, 2000. Figures 2.8, 3.4, 5.28, 18.10, W5.32, W5.6.

- Berg D. *Advanced Clinical Skills and Physical Diagnosis.* Blackwell Science Ltd., 1999. Figures 7.10, 7.12, 7.13, 7.2, 7.3, 7.7, 7.8, 7.9, 8.1, 8.2, 8.4, 8.5, 9.2, 10.2, 11.3, 11.5, 12.6.

- Cuschieri A, Hennessy TPJ, Greenhalgh RM, Rowley DA, Grace PA. *Clinical Surgery.* Osney Mead: Blackwell Science Ltd, 1996. Figures 13.19, 18.22, 18.33.

- Gillespie SH, Bamford K. *Medical Microbiology and Infection at a Glance.* Osney Mead: Blackwell Science Ltd, 2000. Figures 20, 23.

- Ginsberg L. *Lecture Notes on Neurology, 7th Edition.* Osney Mead: Blackwell Science Ltd, 1999. Figures 12.3, 18.3, 18.3b.

- Elliott T, Hastings M, Desselberger U. *Lecture Notes on Medical Microbiology, 3rd Edition.* Osney Mead: Blackwell Science Ltd, 1997. Figures 2, 5, 7, 8, 9, 11, 12, 14, 15, 16, 17, 19, 20, 25, 26, 27, 29, 30, 34, 35, 52.

- Mehta AB, Hoffbrand AV. *Haematology at a Glance.* Osney Mead: Blackwell Science Ltd, 2000. Figures 22.1, 22.2, 22.3.

Please let us know if your name has been missed or misspelled and we will be happy to make the update in the next edition.

PREFACE TO THE 3RD EDITION

We were very pleased with the overwhelmingly positive student feedback for the 2nd edition of our *Underground Clinical Vignettes* series. Well over 100,000 copies of the UCV books are in print and have been used by students all over the world.

Over the last two years we have accumulated and incorporated **over a thousand "updates"** and improvements suggested by you, our readers, including:

- many additions of specific boards and wards testable content

- deletions of redundant and overlapping cases

- reordering and reorganization of all cases in both series

- a new master index by case name in each Atlas

- correction of a few factual errors

- diagnosis and treatment updates

- addition of 5–20 new cases in every book

- and the addition of clinical exam photographs within *UCV— Anatomy*

And most important of all, the third edition sets now include two brand new **COLOR ATLAS** supplements, one for each Clinical Vignette series.

- The *UCV–Basic Science Color Atlas* (*Step 1*) includes over 250 color plates, divided into gross pathology, microscopic pathology (histology), hematology, and microbiology (smears).

- The *UCV–Clinical Science Color Atlas* (*Step 2*) has over 125 color plates, including patient images, dermatology, and funduscopy.

Each atlas image is descriptively captioned and linked to its corresponding Step 1 case, Step 2 case, and/or Step 2 MiniCase.

How Atlas Links Work:

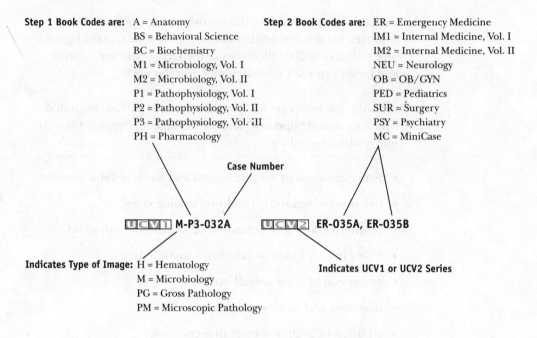

Step 1 Book Codes are:
- A = Anatomy
- BS = Behavioral Science
- BC = Biochemistry
- M1 = Microbiology, Vol. I
- M2 = Microbiology, Vol. II
- P1 = Pathophysiology, Vol. I
- P2 = Pathophysiology, Vol. II
- P3 = Pathophysiology, Vol. III
- PH = Pharmacology

Step 2 Book Codes are:
- ER = Emergency Medicine
- IM1 = Internal Medicine, Vol. I
- IM2 = Internal Medicine, Vol. II
- NEU = Neurology
- OB = OB/GYN
- PED = Pediatrics
- SUR = Surgery
- PSY = Psychiatry
- MC = MiniCase

Case Number

UCV1 M-P3-032A   UCV2 ER-035A, ER-035B

Indicates Type of Image:
- H = Hematology
- M = Microbiology
- PG = Gross Pathology
- PM = Microscopic Pathology

Indicates UCV1 or UCV2 Series

- If the Case number (032, 035, etc.) is not followed by a letter, then there is only one image. Otherwise A, B, C, D indicate up to 4 images.

Bold Faced Links: In order to give you access to the largest number of images possible, we have chosen to cross link the Step 1 and 2 series.

- If the link is bold-faced this indicates that the link is direct (i.e., Step 1 Case with the Basic Science Step 1 Atlas link).

- If the link is not bold-faced this indicates that the link is indirect (Step 1 case with Clinical Science Step 2 Atlas link or vice versa).

We have also implemented a few structural changes upon your request:

- Each current and future edition of our popular *First Aid for the USMLE Step 1* (Appleton & Lange/McGraw-Hill) and *First Aid for the USMLE Step 2* (Appleton & Lange/McGraw-Hill) book will be linked to the corresponding UCV case.

- We eliminated UCV → First Aid links as they frequently become out of date, as the *First Aid* books are revised yearly.

- The Color Atlas is also specially designed for quizzing—captions are descriptive and do not give away the case name directly.

We hope the updated UCV series will remain a unique and well-integrated study tool that provides compact clinical correlations to basic science information. They are designed to be easy and fun (comparatively) to read, and helpful for both licensing exams and the wards.

We invite your corrections and suggestions for the fourth edition of these books. For the first submission of each factual correction or new vignette that is selected for inclusion in the fourth edition, you will receive a personal acknowledgment in the revised book. If you submit over 20 high-quality corrections, additions or new vignettes we will also consider **inviting you to become a "Contributor" on the book of your choice**. If you are interested in becoming a potential "Contributor" or "Author" on a future UCV book, or working with our team in developing additional books, please also e-mail us your CV/resume.

We prefer that you submit corrections or suggestions via electronic mail to **UCVteam@yahoo.com**. Please include "Underground Vignettes" as the subject of your message. If you do not have access to e-mail, use the following mailing address: Blackwell Publishing, Attn: UCV Editors, 350 Main Street, Malden, MA 02148, USA.

Vikas Bhushan
Vishal Pall
Tao Le
October 2001

HOW TO USE THIS BOOK

This series was originally developed to address the increasing number of clinical vignette questions on medical examinations, including the USMLE Step 1 and Step 2. It is also designed to supplement and complement the popular *First Aid for the USMLE Step 1* (Appleton & Lange/McGraw Hill) and *First Aid for the USMLE Step 2* (Appleton & Lange/McGraw Hill).

Each UCV 1 book uses a series of approximately 100 **"supra-prototypical" cases as a way to condense testable facts and associations**. The clinical vignettes in this series are designed to incorporate as many testable facts as possible into a cohesive and memorable clinical picture. The vignettes represent composites drawn from general and specialty textbooks, reference books, thousands of USMLE style questions and the personal experience of the authors and reviewers.

Although each case tends to present all the signs, symptoms, and diagnostic findings for a particular illness, **patients generally will not present with such a "complete" picture either clinically or on a medical examination**. Cases are not meant to simulate a potential real patient or an exam vignette. All the **boldfaced "buzzwords" are for learning purposes** and are not necessarily expected to be found in any one patient with the disease.

Definitions of selected important terms are placed within the vignettes in (SMALL CAPS) in parentheses. Other parenthetical remarks often refer to the pathophysiology or mechanism of disease. The format should also help students learn to present cases succinctly during oral "bullet" presentations on clinical rotations. The cases are meant to serve as a condensed review, not as a primary reference. The information provided in this book has been prepared with a great deal of thought and careful research. This book should not, however, be considered as your sole source of information. Corrections, suggestions and submissions of new cases are encouraged and will be acknowledged and incorporated when appropriate in future editions.

ABBREVIATIONS

5-ASA	5-aminosalicylic acid
ABGs	arterial blood gases
ABVD	adriamycin/bleomycin/vincristine/dacarbazine
ACE	angiotensin-converting enzyme
ACTH	adrenocorticotropic hormone
ADH	antidiuretic hormone
AFP	alpha fetal protein
AI	aortic insufficiency
AIDS	acquired immunodeficiency syndrome
ALL	acute lymphocytic leukemia
ALT	alanine transaminase
AML	acute myelogenous leukemia
ANA	antinuclear antibody
ARDS	adult respiratory distress syndrome
ASD	atrial septal defect
ASO	anti-streptolysin O
AST	aspartate transaminase
AV	arteriovenous
BE	barium enema
BP	blood pressure
BUN	blood urea nitrogen
CAD	coronary artery disease
CALLA	common acute lymphoblastic leukemia antigen
CBC	complete blood count
CHF	congestive heart failure
CK	creatine kinase
CLL	chronic lymphocytic leukemia
CML	chronic myelogenous leukemia
CMV	cytomegalovirus
CNS	central nervous system
COPD	chronic obstructive pulmonary disease
CPK	creatine phosphokinase
CSF	cerebrospinal fluid
CT	computed tomography
CVA	cerebrovascular accident
CXR	chest x-ray
DIC	disseminated intravascular coagulation
DIP	distal interphalangeal
DKA	diabetic ketoacidosis
DM	diabetes mellitus
DTRs	deep tendon reflexes
DVT	deep venous thrombosis

EBV	Epstein–Barr virus
ECG	electrocardiography
Echo	echocardiography
EF	ejection fraction
EGD	esophagogastroduodenoscopy
EMG	electromyography
ERCP	endoscopic retrograde cholangiopancreatography
ESR	erythrocyte sedimentation rate
FEV	forced expiratory volume
FNA	fine needle aspiration
FTA-ABS	fluorescent treponemal antibody absorption
FVC	forced vital capacity
GFR	glomerular filtration rate
GH	growth hormone
GI	gastrointestinal
GM-CSF	granulocyte macrophage colony stimulating factor
GU	genitourinary
HAV	hepatitis A virus
hcG	human chorionic gonadotrophin
HEENT	head, eyes, ears, nose, and throat
HIV	human immunodeficiency virus
HLA	human leukocyte antigen
HPI	history of present illness
HR	heart rate
HRIG	human rabies immune globulin
HS	hereditary spherocytosis
ID/CC	identification and chief complaint
IDDM	insulin-dependent diabetes mellitus
Ig	immunoglobulin
IGF	insulin-like growth factor
IM	intramuscular
JVP	jugular venous pressure
KUB	kidneys/ureter/bladder
LDH	lactate dehydrogenase
LES	lower esophageal sphincter
LFTs	liver function tests
LP	lumbar puncture
LV	left ventricular
LVH	left ventricular hypertrophy
Lytes	electrolytes
MCHC	mean corpuscular hemoglobin concentration
MCV	mean corpuscular volume
MEN	multiple endocrine neoplasia

MGUS	monoclonal gammopathy of undetermined significance
MHC	major histocompatibility complex
MI	myocardial infarction
MOPP	mechlorethamine/vincristine (Oncovorin)/procarbazine/prednisone
MR	magnetic resonance (imaging)
NHL	non-Hodgkin's lymphoma
NIDDM	non-insulin-dependent diabetes mellitus
NPO	nil per os (nothing by mouth)
NSAID	nonsteroidal anti-inflammatory drug
PA	posteroanterior
PIP	proximal interphalangeal
PBS	peripheral blood smear
PE	physical exam
PFTs	pulmonary function tests
PMI	point of maximal intensity
PMN	polymorphonuclear leukocyte
PT	prothrombin time
PTCA	percutaneous transluminal angioplasty
PTH	parathyroid hormone
PTT	partial thromboplastin time
PUD	peptic ulcer disease
RBC	red blood cell
RPR	rapid plasma reagin
RR	respiratory rate
RS	Reed–Sternberg (cell)
RV	right ventricular
RVH	right ventricular hypertrophy
SBFT	small bowel follow-through
SIADH	syndrome of inappropriate secretion of ADH
SLE	systemic lupus erythematosus
STD	sexually transmitted disease
TFTs	thyroid function tests
tPA	tissue plasminogen activator
TSH	thyroid-stimulating hormone
TIBC	total iron-binding capacity
TIPS	transjugular intrahepatic portosystemic shunt
TPO	thyroid peroxidase
TSH	thyroid-stimulating hormone
TTP	thrombotic thrombocytopenic purpura
UA	urinalysis
UGI	upper GI
US	ultrasound

VDRL	Venereal Disease Research Laboratory
VS	vital signs
VT	ventricular tachycardia
WBC	white blood cell
WPW	Wolff–Parkinson–White (syndrome)
XR	x-ray

ID/CC	A 49-year-old **male** immigrant who is a native of Guam has seen three doctors in his country and tried different therapies for marked, **progressive weakness** of his hands and arms, **difficulty speaking**, muscle wasting in both hands, and troublesome **involuntary muscle contractions** (FASCICULATIONS).
HPI	He has no history of sensory symptoms, bladder or bowel dysfunction, fever, exanthem, dog bites, vaccinations, or spinal or cranial trauma.
PE	Lower motor neuron signs: **bilateral wasting of hands**, deep tendon reflexes absent in upper limbs, **muscle weakness, fasciculations**; upper motor neuron signs: positive Babinski's sign, stiffness and spasticity of upper limbs; normal fundus, sensory system, and cranial nerves.
Labs	LP: **CSF normal. Slightly elevated CK**; normal TSH, T_3, and T_4 levels; normal serum calcium and glucose. EMG: partial innervation with abnormal spontaneous activity in resting muscle and reduction in motor units under voluntary control.
Imaging	CT/MR, brain: **brain normal**.
Micro Pathology	Nonspecific atrophy on muscle biopsy.
Treatment	Largely supportive; disease is progressive and fatal.
Discussion	Also known as **Lou Gehrig's disease**, amyotrophic lateral sclerosis (ALS) is a slowly progressive, generalized motor muscle paralysis involving both upper and lower motor neurons.

ID/CC	A **60-year-old** male presents with **speech difficulties**.
HPI	The patient developed this difficulty following a **left-sided stroke** from which he is currently recovering. He is a **diabetic** who has been on insulin for 10 years, and he is also a **chronic smoker**.
PE	Speech **lacks fluency**; patient has difficulty **finding certain words** and sometimes **produces wrong word; comprehension is well preserved**, as are higher mental functions; ability to repeat is better than spontaneous speech; associated recovering right-sided aphasia noted; motor weakness of right upper and lower limbs with exaggerated deep tendon reflexes and right-sided Babinski's reflex.
Labs	Elevated blood glucose; remainder of tests normal.
Imaging	CT: **infarct in region of left frontoparietal cortex**.
Treatment	**Speech therapy** in addition to physiotherapy for stroke; long-term low-dose **aspirin**.
Discussion	This patient has Broca's dysphasia (expressive, nonfluent) with an associated right hemiplegia. The brain damage causing this condition is believed to involve the **dominant inferior frontal gyrus** (BROCA'S AREA). In contrast to patients with Wernicke's aphasia, patients with Broca's aphasia have insight into their condition and are thus at high risk for depression.

ID/CC	A 20-year-old male is brought to the ER after falling from a ladder.
HPI	He fell vertically so that his head hit the ground first. Despite the injury, he is conscious and **does not report any neurologic deficit**, only severe pain in his neck.
PE	**No neurologic deficit found** on clinical examination.
Imaging	XR, cervical spine: **burst fracture of atlas** (JEFFERSON FRACTURE) with ring broken into four pieces.
Treatment	Inherently unstable fracture requiring halo jacket immobilization and fusion if nonunion occurs.
Discussion	The most common mechanism of injury in patients with Jefferson fracture is axial loading. Other cervical spine injuries include **atlantoaxial fracture dislocation**, more frequently associated with neurologic deficit; displacement is commonly anterior, and treatment consists of **skull traction** followed by **immobilization**. A **violent flexion-compression** force may result in a **sudden prolapse of the nucleus pulposus** of the cervical disk into the vertebral canal, producing quadriplegia; here an **early decompression** is required.

ID/CC A **70-year-old male** presents with dull, aching **pain in both calves after moderate exercise**.

HPI The symptoms started a few months ago, typically developing after the patient walked 300 to 400 yards; **symptoms were relieved after a few minutes' rest or when the patient sat down and stooped forward** (pseudoclaudication). In addition to the pain, the patient has experienced numbness in his thighs. He has had no sphincter disturbance but has had **low back pain for many years**.

PE Spinal exam reveals **loss of lumbar lordosis** and reduced flexion and extension of lumbar spine; tone, power, and coordination in lower limbs normal; **reflexes in lower limbs symmetrical but reduced compared to upper limbs**; plantar reflexes flexor; peripheral arterial pulses **present** both at rest and after exercise.

Labs Lab parameters normal.

Imaging XR, lumbar spine: lumbar spondylosis with marked osteophyte formation. CT, spine: **lumbar spinal canal stenosis confirmed**.

Treatment Surgery requiring laminectomy at various levels.

Discussion A number of mechanisms may lead to lumbar canal stenosis, including osteoarthritis with hypertrophy of the facet joints, disk prolapse, surgery, spondylolisthesis, Paget's disease, neoplasia, and infection; any of these conditions may be superimposed on a congenitally narrow spinal canal. The anteroposterior diameter of the cord is narrowed during extension, which tends to compromise the blood supply of the cord, resulting in the development of symptoms; stooping forward does the reverse and therefore relieves symptoms.

ID/CC A 40-year-old male complains of the **"worst headache of his life"** and **double vision**.

HPI He has been **projectile vomiting**. He has no history of fever or neck stiffness.

PE **Papilledema on funduscopic exam; right eye deviated laterally and downward** (due to right third cranial nerve palsy); other cranial nerves normal; no meningeal signs noted; motor system examination normal.

Labs Routine laboratory tests normal.

Imaging Angio, cerebral: posterior communicating (PCOM) artery aneurysm. CT, head: enhancing mass impinging over right third nerve.

Treatment Endovascular or neurosurgical clipping of aneurysm.

Discussion **Congenital berry aneurysms** are associated with **polycystic kidney disease** and **arteriovenous malformation**; they may rupture (during sexual activity, weight lifting, straining) and cause **subarachnoid hemorrhage**.

ID/CC	A 14-year-old white **male** comes into the emergency room because of **projectile vomiting** and a severe **headache**.
HPI	He has a history of unexplained **short stature** and **polyuria**.
PE	**Papilledema and optic disk swelling** (due to increased intracranial pressure) on funduscopic exam; confusion; visual field testing reveals **bitemporal hemianopia**; no other focal neurologic signs; no neurocutaneous markers or meningeal signs.
Imaging	XR, skull: **enlarged sella turcica**. CT/MR: **enhancing**, cystic, multilobulated **suprasellar mass with ring calcification**; hydrocephalus (due to obstruction of foramen of Monro and aqueduct of Sylvius).
Gross Pathology	Cystic mass with concentric areas of calcification.
Micro Pathology	Mixture of squamous epithelial elements and delicate reticular stroma; gliosis seen at periphery; cholesterol-rich cystic fluid.
Treatment	Surgical removal; radiotherapy.
Discussion	Craniopharyngioma is the **most common supratentorial brain tumor in children** and is embryologically derived from **Rathke's pouch remnants**. It is a common cause of growth retardation, diabetes insipidus (compression of pituitary), bitemporal hemianopia (compression of optic chiasm), and headache (obstructive hydrocephalus). It shows a bimodal age distribution with a second peak in the fifth decade.
Atlas Link	UCV1 PG-P3-006

ID/CC A 62-year-old man is brought to his family doctor because of rapidly progressive loss of cognitive function (DEMENTIA) and excessive **somnolence**.

HPI Five years ago, he received a **corneal transplant**. His wife states that she has seen a definite **change in his personality** over the past year.

PE **Dementia; myoclonic fasciculations**; normal funduscopic exam; no other focal neurologic signs.

Labs LP: **normal CSF profile**. EEG: bursts of high-voltage slow-wave activity and slow background.

Imaging CT, head: ventricular enlargement and cerebral atrophy. MR, brain: increased signal intensity in affected areas. PET, brain: areas of diminished glucose metabolism.

Micro Pathology Brain biopsy shows amyloid deposition, **spongiform degeneration**, decrease in neurons of cerebral cortex, and astrocytic proliferation; no inflammatory changes seen.

Treatment Usually fatal; vidarabine and amantadine are being tried.

Discussion A **subacute spongiform encephalopathy** with a very long incubation period, Creutzfeldt–Jakob disease is presumably caused by a **slow virus** or **prion** and transmitted via corneal transplants, **dura mater allografts**, contaminated cadaveric growth hormone, or neurosurgical contamination. Lithium overdose may mimic signs and symptoms.

CREUTZFELDT–JAKOB DISEASE

ID/CC A 35-year-old woman known to have rheumatic mitral stenosis awakens in the morning to find the **right side of her body paralyzed**.

HPI The patient also complains of **palpitations**. She has no history of fever, neck stiffness, vomiting, headache, or transient ischemic attacks (TIAs).

PE VS: no fever; irregularly irregular pulse. PE: dense **right-sided hemiplegia; brisk reflexes on right side; right-sided Babinski** (EXTENSOR PLANTAR RESPONSE) **present**; fundus normal; loud S1; apical mid-diastolic murmur and opening snap.

Labs ECG: presence of atrial fibrillation confirmed in addition to P-mitrale. Blood culture sterile; routine lab tests normal; clotting time, bleeding time, and PT normal.

Imaging Echo: left atrial thrombus. CT: scan performed after 24 hours reveals **infarct in posterior limb of left internal capsule**.

Treatment Start heparin after follow-up; therapy guided with PT; digoxin for management of atrial fibrillation; valvuloplasty or valve replacement after resolution of left atrial thrombus.

Discussion Mitral stenosis with atrial fibrillation predisposes to thromboembolism.

ID/CC	A **65-year-old** white **male** develops **sudden severe headache** and **right-sided hemiplegia**.
HPI	The patient is a **known hypertensive** and takes his medication irregularly; he now has both **urinary and fecal incontinence**.
PE	VS: **severe hypertension** (BP 210/180); no fever. PE: dense right-sided **hemiplegia**; funduscopic exam reveals presence of **papilledema** in addition to **hypertensive retinopathy**; right-sided **Babinski**; eyes deviated toward left; no meningeal signs present.
Labs	Routine labs normal; LP not done, since intracranial pressure (ICP) raised.
Imaging	CT, head: **focal hemorrhage** in left putamen region of basal ganglia.
Gross Pathology	Autopsy: mass of blood dissecting through parenchyma into deep structures of brain and ventricles.
Micro Pathology	Hypertensive changes seen in addition to putamenal hemorrhage; hyaline arteriolosclerosis; lipohyalinosis; Charcot–Bouchard aneurysms.
Treatment	Supportive management to **reduce ICP** and **blood pressure**.
Discussion	Bleeding is most often caused by hypertension. In the presence of moderate to severe hypertension, **small penetrating arterioles** may rupture deep within the brain, causing a **hematoma** that displaces brain structures. Common sites are the **putamen, thalamus, pons**, and **cerebellum**.

CVA, HYPERTENSIVE

ID/CC	A 19-year-old female Olympic horseback rider is brought into the emergency room with **headache, confusion, weakness of the left side of her body, blurred vision, and projectile vomiting**.
HPI	Three hours ago, she hit the right side of her head when she fell from a horse during a training exercise. She **lost consciousness** for 1 minute and then appeared to have **recovered completely** before presenting with the symptomatology (LUCID INTERVAL).
PE	VS: BP mildly elevated; **bradycardia**. PE: **papilledema**; right-sided **mydriasis**; efferent pupillary reflex abnormality on right side; **deviation of right eyeball outward and downward** (RIGHT CN III PALSY); left-sided weakness; brisk reflexes on left side; **extensor plantar response** on left side.
Imaging	CT/MR, head: right temporal bone fracture; right-sided **lens-shaped** (convex) **hyperdense extra-axial fluid collection**.
Gross Pathology	**Collection of blood between dura mater and skull** with mass effect.
Treatment	Emergent surgical evacuation.
Discussion	The results of arterial bleeding (rupture of **middle meningeal artery**) are usually associated with skull fracture. Classically, the patient loses consciousness immediately after head injury but regains consciousness and remains asymptomatic for a variable period of time before symptoms worsen.
Atlas Link	UCVI PG-P3-010

EPIDURAL HEMATOMA

ID/CC	A 19-year-old male visits his orthopedist because of a **wide-based gait** (ATAXIC GAIT), congenital **clubfoot**, and **abnormal lateral curvature of the spine** (SCOLIOSIS).
HPI	For the past several years, he has had **increasing difficulty walking**; the process began subtly, but he is now incapable of participating in sports. He also complains of a **progressive diminution of vision**.
PE	VS: **arrhythmia; tachycardia**. PE: bilateral concentric contraction of visual fields on visual field testing; findings suggestive of **retinitis pigmentosa** on retinal exam; scoliosis of thoracic spine; pes cavus deformity of right foot; diminished sensation in stocking-glove distribution; **proprioceptive sensory loss; areflexia; ataxia** of limbs; **Babinski's** sign; **forceful pulse; prominent JVP; sustained apical impulse; S4** (due to hypertrophic cardiomyopathy).
Labs	ECG: left ventricular hypertrophy; inverted T waves.
Imaging	Echo: evidence of hypertrophic obstructive cardiomyopathy.
Micro Pathology	Marked loss of cells in posterior root ganglia and degeneration of peripheral sensory fibers; posterior and lateral columns of CNS also affected.
Treatment	No treatment available.
Discussion	The most common hereditary ataxia, Friedreich's ataxia is an **autosomal-recessive** disorder due to a defective gene on chromosome 9.

FRIEDREICH'S ATAXIA

ID/CC	A 60-year-old white male complains of **headache** that is **worse in the morning** along with occasional **nausea and vomiting** for 6 weeks.
HPI	One day prior to presentation, he had an isolated **grand mal seizure**.
PE	Bilateral papilledema; loss of recent memory; **brisk deep tendon reflexes** on right side; **Babinski** on right side.
Imaging	CT/MR: **irregular enhancing left-sided mass** with **necrotic center; mass effect** and **surrounding edema**.
Gross Pathology	Hemorrhagic and necrotic tumor mass infiltrating left parietal lobe.
Micro Pathology	Biopsy reveals presence of anaplastic cells with pleomorphism and endothelial proliferation; **foci of necrosis** surrounded by palisading.
Treatment	Surgical resection; chemotherapy; radiotherapy.
Discussion	Astrocytomas are graded according to differentiation; the **highest grade** (grade IV) **is glioblastoma multiforme**. It carries a poor prognosis.
Atlas Links	U C V 1 PG-P3-012, PM-P3-012

GLIOBLASTOMA MULTIFORME

ID/CC A 38-year-old male visits his family doctor complaining of **symmetric muscle weakness** that started **distally in his legs and ascended gradually**, now involving the trunk and arms.

HPI One week ago he suffered from **diarrhea and fever** and was diagnosed with and treated for *Campylobacter* **enteritis**.

PE **Symmetrical** proximal muscle **weakness** and **flaccidity** in lower limbs; absent deep tendon reflexes; normal sensory exam; normal cranial nerves.

Labs Elevated gamma globulin. LP: **increased CSF protein concentration without cellular increase**; normal glucose. Nonreactive VDRL; **decreased nerve conduction velocity** indicative of **demyelination** on electrophysiologic studies.

Treatment Plasmapheresis; intensive care and respiratory support.

Discussion Guillain-Barré syndrome is a common cause of **polyneuropathy** in adults that is usually **preceded by** GI or respiratory **infection** or by specific illnesses such as Epstein–Barr, *Campylobacter* enteritis, and cytomegalovirus infection. **Respiratory paralysis** may occur, necessitating **mechanical ventilation**.

GUILLAIN–BARRÉ SYNDROME

ID/CC	A 50-year-old male presents to the emergency room with **wild, flinging movements of his left arm and leg**.
HPI	He has been diagnosed with **diabetes and hypertension** but has taken his medications only irregularly. He is also a **chronic smoker**.
PE	Uncontrolled, violent, rapid flinging movements of left arm and leg; remainder of neurologic exam normal.
Labs	Lab tests reveal elevated blood glucose.
Imaging	CT (done at 48 hours): infarct in right **subthalamic nucleus**.
Treatment	Phenothiazines and dopamine antagonists such as sulpiride and tetrabenazine may be of help.
Discussion	Hemiballismus is characterized by forceful, flinging, and violent movements, primarily of the proximal parts of the limbs of one side of the body, that disappear during sleep. The most common etiology is that of a vascular event in the contralateral subthalamic nucleus; other causes include an expanding arteriovenous malformation, trauma, tumor, and multiple sclerosis. Most cases resolve spontaneously within 6 to 8 weeks; however, surgery may be indicated in cases of intractable involuntary movements.

ID/CC	A **42-year-old** male presents with **depression**, poor memory, and **jerking movements** of the limbs and fingers.
HPI	His **father died of a similar** condition in which the symptoms progressively worsened, proceeding to dementia until his death at the age of 50.
PE	**Chorea**; psychiatric evaluation reveals **cognitive impairment** (inattention and poor concentration without memory loss) and depression; no other focal neurologic deficit found.
Labs	Routine laboratory tests unremarkable.
Imaging	MR, brain: degeneration of **caudate nucleus**. CT, brain: cerebral atrophy.
Gross Pathology	Loss of brain mass with striking **atrophy of caudate nucleus** and, less strikingly, putamen; secondary loss of neurons in globus pallidus; cortical atrophy most commonly occurs in frontal lobe.
Micro Pathology	Degeneration of spiny GABAergic neurons in the striatum leads to a net loss of inhibitory signals from the striatum.
Treatment	No specific treatment available; supportive and symptomatic treatment; genetic counseling with regard to future offspring.
Discussion	Huntington's chorea is an **autosomal-dominant** disease whose gene locus is on chromosome 4. It is caused by expansion of a **trinucleotide repeat** (CAG) within the Huntington gene; expansion of the trinucleotide repeat leads to greater frequency of disease in successive generations (GENETIC ANTICIPATION). The onset of the disease is typically between 30 and 50 years of age, progressing to death within 15 to 20 years.

ID/CC	A 25-year-old male is brought to a neurologist with complaints of **inability to see on one side**.
HPI	Two months ago he suffered **right eye optic neuritis**, but his vision has significantly improved since then, although it is not completely normal.
PE	On lateral gaze in either direction, one eye does not adduct and the other has **nystagmus** on abduction (finding characteristic of bilateral internuclear ophthalmoplegia); funduscopy reveals temporal pallor of right disk (due to atrophy of papillomacular fibers); visual field testing reveals right paracentral scotoma; **flexion of neck produces an electrical sensation that runs down back and into legs** (LHERMITTE'S SIGN; suggests intramedullary disease of cervical cord).
Labs	LP: specific increase in CSF IgG concentration. Agarose electrophoresis reveals oligoclonal bands in IgG region of CSF. Evoked-potential studies of visual, auditory, and somatosensory pathways indicate impaired responses.
Imaging	MR, brain (T2W): investigation of choice; reveals **multiple, discrete, white-matter plaques**.
Gross Pathology	Sharply defined areas of gray discoloration (PLAQUES) of white matter that occur particularly frequently around the ventricles and in the corpus callosum.
Micro Pathology	Active plaques show evidence of myelin breakdown, lipid-laden macrophages, loss of oligodendrocytes, and relative preservation of axons; lymphocytes and mononuclear cells prominent at edges of plaques.
Treatment	Beta-interferon; immunosuppression (corticosteroids, azathioprine, cyclosporine), but success has been modest.
Discussion	The following are suggestive of multiple sclerosis: (1) optic neuritis, whose early signs include diminished visual acuity, central or paracentral scotoma, hyperemia and edema of the optic disk, and a defective pupillary reaction to light; (2) internuclear ophthalmoplegia (due to demyelination of the medial longitudinal fasciculus); and (3) Lhermitte's sign.

ID/CC A 15-year-old male is brought to a physician by his parents for an evaluation of recently observed **overindulgence in sexual activities**.

HPI The parents also report that the patient's behavior has recently changed markedly from **aggressive to extremely placid**; directed questioning reveals that he has now started **exploring things orally** and has developed a voracious appetite. He suffered from **herpes simplex encephalitis** a few months ago. There is no history of prior psychiatric illness in the patient or in the family.

PE Patient is in excellent health and is apparently unconcerned about his illness, displaying no reaction to parents' complaints; when physician attempts to shake his hand, patient begins to orally explore it; on seeing a nurse in doctor's room, he starts to masturbate.

Imaging MR/CT, head: **bilateral temporal lobe and amygdala damage**.

Treatment No specific treatment available.

Discussion Klüver–Bucy syndrome is a syndrome of **hyperphagia, hypersexuality, placidity, and hyperorality**. In experimental animals, it results from **bilateral removal of the amygdala**; in humans, an incomplete picture is generally seen secondary to extensive temporal lobe damage, as may occur during herpes simplex encephalitis or in degenerative or post-traumatic brain damage.

ID/CC	A **6-year-old** male is brought to the emergency room with acute-onset **projectile vomiting**, severe headache, and blurring of vision.
HPI	The patient reports **unsteadiness of gait** that has progressively worsened over the past 2 months. He has no history of seizures, fever, or neck stiffness.
PE	**Papilledema**; no meningeal signs; nystagmus in all directions of gaze; truncal ataxia; cranial nerves normal.
Labs	CBC: mild anemia.
Imaging	CT/MR, brain: homogeneous, enhancing **mass in cerebellar vermis** compressing and filling fourth ventricle; **dilated third and lateral ventricles** (due to obstructive hydrocephalus).
Gross Pathology	Soft, well-circumscribed, light-grayish mass on cerebellar vermis.
Micro Pathology	Once intracranial pressure (ICP) is controlled, CSF on lumbar puncture shows malignant cells; highly malignant tumor characterized by deeply staining nuclei with scant cytoplasm arranged in **pseudorosettes**.
Treatment	Corticosteroids for increased ICP; entire neuraxis irradiation; surgical extirpation; chemotherapy.
Discussion	A common tumor of **childhood** and the most prevalent brain tumor in children less than 7 years of age, medulloblastoma is classified as a primitive neuroectodermal tumor (PNET).
Atlas Link	⬜C⬜1 PG-P3-018

ID/CC A 40-year-old **man** complains that "the whole room seems to be spinning" (VERTIGO) while also experiencing ringing in the ears (TINNITUS) and nausea.

HPI The patient also complains of a **sense of fullness** in his ears and adds that his **hearing has progressively diminished** over the past few years. His symptoms were initially **unilateral but have now become bilateral**. His illness has run a course of **remissions and relapses**. He denies any weakness of the limbs and has no history of ear discharge or trauma.

PE VS: normal. PE: anxious; neurologic exam normal; caloric tests bilaterally normal.

Labs Pure-tone audiometry reveals **sensorineural hearing loss** that is more marked for **lower frequencies**; loudness recruitment present; short-increment sensitivity index (SISI) shows high score; VDRL negative.

Imaging MR/CT, head: normal (performed to rule out internal auditory canal pathology).

Micro Pathology **Gross distention of the endolymphatic system** (ENDOLYMPHATIC HYDROPS)

Treatment No specific treatment; symptomatic relief with **vestibular suppressants, diuretics**, and low-sodium diet. Surgical intervention is controversial.

Discussion Ménière's is a disease of the inner ear characterized by **acute onset** and **recurrent attacks of vertigo**; it is often associated with nausea and vomiting **together with diminished hearing and tinnitus**. Although the exact etiology is unknown, endolymphatic hydrops (due to excess of endolymph in the scala media) has been linked to obstruction of resorption, defective membrane exchange, and increased endolymph inflow (secondary to allergy, vasomotor factors, or retained sodium and water).

MÉNIÈRE'S DISEASE

ID/CC	A 60-year-old **woman** is seen with complaints of having difficulty walking and two episodes of **involuntary hand jerking** (PARTIAL SEIZURE).
HPI	Her attendant reveals that over the past few months her **memory has deteriorated**. She has slow mentation and **urinary incontinence**. She is not diabetic or hypertensive.
PE	Funduscopy reveals papilledema; tone of lower limbs increased and strength reduced (SPASTIC PARAPARESIS); deep tendon reflexes exaggerated; bilateral Babinski.
Labs	Routine laboratory tests normal.
Imaging	XR, skull: **hyperostosis** of left parietal bone and sagittal suture. CT (with contrast): left parietal **parasagittal tumor**. MR (gadolinium): **intense tumor enhancement; dural extension** and invasion into superior sagittal sinus.
Gross Pathology	Irregular, firm, **gritty mass arising superficially, indenting and compressing brain but not invading it**.
Micro Pathology	**Whorling pattern** of meningothelial cells with regular, oval nuclei, indistinct cytoplasm, and **psammoma bodies**.
Treatment	Surgical resection; radiation for unresectable cases.
Discussion	Meningioma is a primary intracranial neoplasm arising from cells of the **arachnoid granulations**; it is characterized by **slow growth, benign behavior, and expansile rather than infiltrative growth**. Common sites involved include the cerebral convexity, parasagittal area (as in this case), sphenoid wing, olfactory groove, cerebellopontine angle, foramen magnum, and spinal cord. The tumor is usually solitary, is more common in women, and is found in middle and later ages. Multiple meningiomas may be found in patients with neurofibromatosis type 2.
Atlas Links	UCV1 PM-P3-020, PG-P3-020

ID/CC	A 59-year-old white female presents with a **severe, dull retro-orbital headache**, vomiting, and **diplopia**.
HPI	She has **smoked** two packs of cigarettes a day for 22 years and has been diagnosed with **lung cancer**.
PE	VS: bradycardia; mild hypertension. PE: **papilledema** (due to increased intracranial pressure); **right pupillary reflex abnormality** in efferent pathway (due to right oculomotor nerve palsy).
Imaging	CT/MR: round, discrete, **ring-enhancing lesion** in right frontal lobe; surrounding vasogenic edema; **shifting of midline structures to left** (> 1-cm shift considered severe).
Micro Pathology	Biopsy shows small cell carcinoma.
Treatment	Consider surgical resection; radiation therapy; dexamethasone (to control intracranial pressure).
Discussion	Blood-borne brain metastases commonly occur in patients with systemic malignancy. Common primary cancers that result in intracranial metastasis are lung, breast, GI, and GU cancer and melanoma.
Atlas Link	UCV1 PM-P3-021

METASTATIC BRAIN TUMOR

ID/CC A **20-year-old woman** complains of **recurrent, throbbing headaches** associated with profound **nausea and light sensitivity**.

HPI She has had similar headaches several times each year since the onset of her menstrual periods. The headaches occur on **one side of her head**. She also reports seeing **"flashing lights"** like lightning moving across her field of vision. **Stress, sleeplessness, and anxiety usually precipitate** these headaches. Her mother suffers from migraine headaches (positive family history).

PE VS: normal. PE: funduscopic exam and visual field testing normal; neurologic exam normal.

Treatment Prophylactic therapy with avoidance of precipitating factors and drugs such as beta-blockers, tricyclic antidepressants, or calcium channel blockers; abortive therapy during acute attacks with NSAIDs, sumatriptan, ergotamine, or transnasal butorphanol.

Discussion Migraine headache is the **second most common** cause of **primary headache** (the most common in the United States is tension headache). In the United States, an estimated **17% of women** and 6% of men are affected by this disorder. The headache is characteristically preceded by a **prodrome** and is **episodic**, gradual in onset, **usually unilateral**, and most commonly in the **temporal area**. Precipitating factors may include menses, fasting, emotional stress, and foods containing tyramine, monosodium glutamate, or nitrites. The cause is unknown but appears to involve variations in cerebral blood flow and serotonergic pathways.

ID/CC	A **36-year-old white** female pays an emergency visit to her ophthalmologist because of **loss of central vision and pain on movement of her left eye** (due to optic neuritis); she also presents with scanning speech and **intention tremor** in the hands.
HPI	Five years ago, she **emigrated** to the United States from **Sweden**. She has been suffering from **recurrent paresthesias in the hands, arms, and legs; weakness in the legs and arms; vertigo**; and **bladder urgency** (multiple unrelated neurologic symptoms). Her family doctor told her she had "hysteria" and recommended psychotherapy.
PE	Diminished visual acuity; central scotoma found on visual field charting; **hyperemia and edema** of left **optic disk**; defective afferent pupillary reaction to light in left eye (MARCUS GUNN PUPIL); **paresis of medial rectus muscle on lateral conjugate gaze but not on convergence** (BILATERAL INTERNUCLEAR OPHTHALMOPLEGIA); **nystagmus** in abducting eye; electrical sensation running down back and into legs produced by neck flexion (LHERMITTE'S SIGN); leg spasticity and increased deep tendon reflexes.
Labs	LP: **marked increase in CSF IgG concentration**; presence of **oligoclonal bands** in IgG region on CSF agarose electrophoresis; CSF otherwise normal. Abnormal visual, auditory, and somatosensory evoked responses.
Imaging	MR, brain: multiple discrete high T2 signal abnormalities in **periventricular** and other white matter areas (especially **corpus callosum**).
Gross Pathology	Pathologic hallmark of disorder consists of distinctive small gray **plaques of demyelination** present in CNS white matter; optic neuritis.
Micro Pathology	Demyelination and gliosis; lipid-laden macrophages.
Treatment	Mainly supportive; corticosteroids; ACTH; azathioprine; cyclophosphamide.
Discussion	Multiple sclerosis is an idiopathic demyelinating disorder whose course is marked by **intermittent remissions and exacerbations**.
Atlas Link	UCV1 PG-P3-023

ID/CC   A 25-year-old **female** has had marked **weakness** and **drooping of the eyelids** (PTOSIS) in the evening for the past 4 weeks; she does not experience any weakness in the morning following a good night's sleep.

HPI   She has also been suffering from **double vision** (DIPLOPIA) at the end of each day.

PE   **Ptosis** develops on sustained elevation of eyelids; **dysphonia** develops as patient is asked to narrate complaints at length; **weakness of forward flexion of head develops after repetitive resistance to force**; patient could not maintain her upper limb in abducted position for more than a minute.

Labs   **Clear-cut improvement in strength with edrophonium** administration. EMG: progressive decrement in voltage during repetitive, low-frequency stimulation of motor nerve. **Positive serum titer of antibodies to acetylcholine receptors**.

Treatment   Acetylcholinesterase inhibitors (pyridostigmine); prednisone; thymectomy; plasmapheresis.

Discussion   Myasthenia gravis is an **autoimmune disease** that is due to the development of specific **antibodies to one or more acetylcholine receptor subunits**, reducing the availability of acetylcholine receptors at the neuromuscular junction. **Thymoma** is present in 20% of cases.

ID/CC	An obese 35-year-old male goes to a clinic because of **distal muscle weakness** in both upper and lower limbs and **gradual diminution of vision**.
HPI	His **father** suffered from a **similar muscular weakness**. The patient also suffers from mental retardation.
PE	**Frontal balding**; typical **facial wasting**; bilateral cataracts; **distal muscle weakness** in both upper and lower limbs; difficulty releasing grip after handshake; **percussion over tongue and thenar eminence reveals myotonia**; mildly reduced deep tendon reflexes; normal sensory exam; moderately **atrophic testicles**; equinovarus deformity of both feet.
Labs	**Decreased plasma IgG**. EMG: myopathic potentials; myotonia.
Imaging	ECG: nonspecific ST-T changes.
Micro Pathology	Muscle biopsy reveals internal nuclei (nuclei in center of the fiber rather than in periphery), type I fiber atrophy, and ring fibers.
Treatment	Phenytoin; carbamazepine; quinidine; procainamide; acetazolamide; surgery required to correct foot deformities.
Discussion	The most common form of muscular dystrophy among **whites**, myotonic dystrophy is transmitted as an **autosomal-dominant** trait. It is associated with a genetic defect that encodes **myotonin protein kinase**; the myotonic dystrophy gene locus has been mapped at chromosome 19q13.3.

MYOTONIC DYSTROPHY

ID/CC	A **5-year-old male** is referred to a specialist by his physician for evaluation of an **abdominal mass** and a recently noticed **left-sided orbital proptosis**.
HPI	His parents complain of weight loss, poor feeding, and a continuous low-grade fever for the past few months.
PE	PE: marked **cachexia**; left-sided orbital proptosis and ecchymoses; large, smooth **intra-abdominal mass palpable**.
Labs	Marked **elevation of urinary catecholamines** and metabolites vanillylmandelic acid (VMA) and homovanillic acid (HVA).
Imaging	CT, abdomen: **intra-abdominal mass arising from and obliterating left adrenal gland**. Nuc (bone scan): metastatic lytic lesion in left orbital region of skull.
Gross Pathology	Solid, round soft-tumor mass obliterating left adrenal gland; **gray on cut surface** showing extensive hemorrhage and necrosis with cyst formation.
Micro Pathology	Anaplastic, small, round-to-oval hyperchromatic cells with scant cytoplasm in sheets and at places forming **Homer–Wright pseudorosettes**; few ganglion cells seen; electron microscopy reveals presence of **neurosecretory granules**.
Treatment	Surgical resection; chemotherapy with cyclophosphamide and adriamycin.
Discussion	Neuroblastoma is a primary malignant neoplasm that arises from immature cells of the adrenal medulla and secretes catecholamines; it usually occurs in children under the age of 5 and presents with an abdominal mass. Neuroblastomas most commonly originate in the adrenal glands but may also arise in the retroperitoneal sympathetic ganglia, pelvis, neck, or posterior mediastinum. Hutchinson's neuroblastoma presents with extensive skull and orbital metastases that produce exophthalmos; metastases to lymph nodes, liver, lung, and bone are common.
Atlas Links	UCV1 PG-P3-026, PM-P3-026

ID/CC   A 60-year-old male is seen by a neurologist for an evaluation of **deteriorating cognitive skills**.

HPI   Over the past few weeks, the patient has stayed in bed and has had urinary and bowel incontinence.

PE   Cognition impaired; impaired ambulation without evidence of primary motor, sensory, or cerebellar dysfunction (GAIT APRAXIA); deep tendon reflexes intact; pupils equal, round, and reactive to light and accommodation; plantars bilaterally flexor; fundus does not reveal any papilledema.

Labs   LP: normal opening pressure. Lab parameters within normal limits.

Imaging   CT: **ventricular enlargement with relatively little cortical atrophy**. Nuc, cisternography: persistent activity of radionuclide in lateral ventricles after 48 hours (**characteristic of normal pressure hydrocephalus**).

Treatment   Insertion of a ventriculoperitoneal shunt.

Discussion   Pseudobulbar palsy is due to bilateral dysfunction of the corticobulbar tracts. In addition to dysphagia, dysarthria, and hyperactive gag reflexes, patients may experience episodes of spontaneous crying or laughter. In most patients, the cause of normal pressure hydrocephalus is not known, although it may follow a subarachnoid hemorrhage or meningitis (sometimes years later). The value of its early diagnosis lies in the fact that it is a **treatable dementia**.

ID/CC	A 46-year-old white male complains to his internist of increasingly severe **headaches upon awakening** of a few months' duration; the headaches persist throughout the afternoon and are mild in the evenings.
HPI	While in the doctor's office, the patient suffers a **seizure** and is brought to the emergency room.
PE	Funduscopy reveals papilledema.
Labs	Normal.
Imaging	CT/MR: large **frontal lobe mass** with focal **nodular calcifications**.
Gross Pathology	Calcified cystic tumor with gelatinous consistency and areas of necrosis and hemorrhage.
Micro Pathology	Tumor has **few anaplastic features**; regular cells aligned smoothly; spherical nuclei with finely granular chromatin, calcifications, and increased vascularity with areas of intratumoral bleeding.
Treatment	Surgical resection/chemotherapy with radiation.
Discussion	Usually low grade but occasionally anaplastic, oligodendrogliomas resemble astrocytomas in most respects but grow more slowly and are **more sensitive to chemotherapy**; calcification is noted in 90% of cases.

ID/CC   A 40-year-old male with a history of **insulin-dependent diabetes mellitus (IDDM)** presents with **tingling, numbness, burning, and aching in the lower legs and feet**.

HPI   The discomfort is particularly prominent at night and is often **relieved by walking**. A hoop over the feet to prevent contact with bedclothes is often helpful. The patient takes **insulin** irregularly.

PE   Mild weakness; mild **distal sensory loss** and **loss of position and vibration sense** in both legs; bilaterally reduced ankle and knee jerks.

Labs   Nerve conduction velocities slowed. EMG: features of **denervation**. Elevated glycosylated hemoglobin levels indicate poor blood sugar control.

Treatment   NSAIDs and carbamazepine effective in reducing discomfort; good glycemic control to slow progression of neuropathy.

Atlas Link   `UCV2` MC-259

ID/CC	A 35-year-old male who has been diagnosed with **multiple sclerosis** visits his physician with complaints of **difficulty swallowing** (DYSPHAGIA) and **nasal regurgitation** of food.
HPI	Six months ago he suffered an attack of retrobulbar neuritis; 2 months ago he developed **spastic weakness of both lower limbs**.
PE	Speech is monotonous, slurred, and high-pitched ("DONALD DUCK" DYSARTHRIA); dribbles from mouth; cannot protrude his **tongue, which lies on the floor of the mouth and is small and spastic**; palatal movements absent; jaw jerk exaggerated; patient is emotionally labile.
Imaging	MR, brain: multiple focal white-matter plaques.
Treatment	General management of multiple sclerosis; no specific treatment available.
Discussion	The common causes of pseudobulbar palsy include bilateral cerebrovascular accidents involving the **internal capsule**, motor neuron disease, and multiple sclerosis.

ID/CC	A 40-year-old male **dies** shortly after being brought to the emergency room with the **"most severe headache of his life."**
HPI	His father died of chronic renal failure at the age of 45.
Imaging	CT, head: **hyperdense blood** in cisterns and sulci.
Gross Pathology	Brain reveals staining of inferior surfaces of brainstem, cerebellum, and cerebral hemispheres with fresh blood due to congenital berry aneurysm rupture; both kidneys reveal polycystic changes; multiple cysts seen in liver.
Discussion	In this case, hemorrhage was caused by a ruptured intracranial aneurysm in a patient with **autosomal-dominant polycystic kidney disease**. Other causes of subarachnoid hemorrhage include AV malformation and trauma.
Atlas Link	ⓊⒸⓋ① PG-P3-031

ID/CC	A 30-year-old black male complains of **constant bifrontal headache** and **blurred vision** of 3 weeks' duration.
HPI	He has had mild intermittent **frontal headaches for the past 8 months** and has become **irritable**; for the past month he has been **extremely drowsy** and often sleeps for 30 hours at a time. Ten months ago, **he fell** from a moving vehicle and **lacerated his scalp**.
PE	**Bilateral papilledema; dilated left pupil**; right spastic hemiparesis; deep tendon reflexes on right side are brisk; **right-sided Babinski**; no meningeal signs present.
Labs	LP contraindicated due to raised intracranial pressure.
Imaging	CT, head: **hyperdense crescentic extra-axial fluid collections (early); hypodense fluid collection with thick membranes (late)**.
Gross Pathology	Old blood encased in thick adherent brown membranes.
Micro Pathology	Outer membrane composed of granulation and fibrous tissue with hemosiderin; inner membrane shows fibrous tissue only.
Treatment	Surgical drainage of hematoma.
Discussion	Subdural hematoma is a traumatic lesion characterized by accumulation of blood between the dura and arachnoid. It is caused by **laceration of the bridging veins** and results in **displacement of the brain** and possible **cerebral herniations**.
Atlas Link	🅄🅒🅥🅘 PG-P3-032

ID/CC A 30-year-old man is referred to a neurologist because of progressive **anesthesia and weakness of both arms, occipital headaches,** and a **stiff gait.**

HPI He has no history of significant trauma in the past.

PE No motor deficits; **lack of pain and temperature sensation in both hands and arms** (due to spinothalamic tract involvement) **but preserved position and tactile sensation** (dorsal columns uninvolved and proprioceptive sensation spared); unimpaired pain and temperature sensation below arms; **thenar muscles** of both hands **atrophied; areflexia in both upper limbs;** brisk deep tendon reflexes in both lower limbs.

Labs Normal.

Imaging MR/CT, spine: **cystic dilatation within central cervical cord.**

Gross Pathology Spinal cord shows **central cavitation** in longitudinal and cleftlike fashion.

Micro Pathology Hydromyelia is lined by ependymal tissue; syringomyelia is not.

Treatment Surgical shunting.

Discussion Syringomyelia may be primary (associated with **Arnold–Chiari malformation**) or acquired (post-traumatic, postinflammatory, tumor-associated).

ID/CC	A **79-year-old** white woman complains of a **throbbing, unilateral headache** that is most severe around her forehead and temples.
HPI	She has had recurrent bouts of **fever** over the past year and also complains of **malaise** and **muscle aches**. She reports some weight loss and occasional **vision problems** in her right eye. She also reports **pain in her mandible when she is eating** (JAW CLAUDICATION).
PE	VS: fever. PE: **nodular enlargement of temporal artery with tenderness.**
Labs	CBC: normal WBC count; mild anemia. **Markedly elevated ESR,** usually > 100 mm/hour.
Gross Pathology	Swollen, cordlike, segmentally nodular temporal artery.
Micro Pathology	**Granulomatous** inflammatory infiltrate of media and adventitia on **temporal artery biopsy**; fragmentation of internal elastic lamina with multinucleated giant cells and fibrotic patches.
Treatment	**Steroids** should be started empirically before biopsy confirmation to **prevent blindness**.
Discussion	Temporal arteritis is the most **common vasculitis** in the United States; it frequently **coexists with polymyalgia rheumatica** and carries a risk of ipsilateral **blindness** due to thrombosis of the **ophthalmic artery**. Diagnosis and treatment are based on clinical grounds, since biopsy is positive in only 60% of cases.
Atlas Link	UCV1 PM-P3-034

ID/CC An 18-year-old man presents with **headache, ataxia**, and progressive loss of vision.

HPI His **father** died of metastatic **bilateral renal cell carcinoma** at a relatively **young** age.

PE **Cerebellar ataxia; nystagmus**; past-pointing and **inability to perform rapid alternating movements** (DYSDIADOCHOKINESIA); funduscopic exam reveals presence of **retinal hemangiomas** and moderate papilledema (due to increased intracranial pressure).

Labs UA: normal (hematuria may signal renal cell carcinoma).

Imaging CT/MR, head: **cerebellar solid/cystic lesion** with **enhancing mural nodule.** CT, abdomen: **renal, hepatic, and pancreatic cysts.**

Gross Pathology **Hemangioblastomas** of cerebellum and retina; tumor occasionally located in medulla or cervical spinal cord.

Treatment Surgical removal of tumor; photocoagulation for treatment of retinal lesions.

Discussion Von Hippel–Lindau disease is a rare **autosomal-dominant** neurocutaneous dysplasia. The gene has been linked to the raf-1 oncogene on chromosome 3 and has a variable penetrance and delayed expression. The condition is **associated with renal cell carcinoma** that is often multifocal or bilateral.

ID/CC A 45-year-old Hispanic female is brought to the gynecologist for an evaluation of a **gross difference in the size of her breasts** of recent origin.

HPI Her medical history is unremarkable. Despite the recent increase in the size of her right breast, she **does not feel any pain and feels only a sensation of fullness**.

PE **Very large mass** with **firm, "wooden-log" consistency** involving almost all of right breast, making it twice the size of opposite breast; **mobile mass**; appears **well circumscribed; collateral bluish veins seen on skin** along with striae; no peau d'orange appearance; no nipple retraction, axillary lymphadenopathy, or hepatomegaly; opposite breast normal.

Imaging US: large, smooth multilobulated mass.

Gross Pathology Large tumor with numerous **cystic spaces on cut section of stroma, producing recesses and longitudinal openings** and causing a leaflike **(phyllodes)** appearance.

Micro Pathology Abundance of normal-looking ducts, acini, and stroma with no signs of cellular atypia and low mitotic index.

Treatment Simple excision.

Discussion A less common benign tumor of breast that is also known as giant fibroadenoma, cystosarcoma phyllodes is a **bulky tumor** that, although usually benign histologically, **may recur** following excision and sometimes undergoes malignant degeneration (5% to 10%). It **rarely metastasizes** to lymph nodes or distant sites.

Atlas Link UCV1 PM-P3-036

ID/CC A 27-year-old **woman** who is **actively training** for a marathon notes a **painful lump** in the upper outer quadrant of her right breast of 2 days' duration.

HPI She has no history of fever and no known family history of breast cancer.

PE **Retraction of overlying skin** in upper outer quadrant of right breast; **indurated lesion** the size of a lemon in same area; axillary lymph nodes not palpable.

Imaging Mammo: **irregular mass** with **focal areas** of **eggshell calcification**.

Gross Pathology Yellowish, fatty fluid on aspiration.

Micro Pathology Excisional biopsy shows localized area of **granulation tissue** within which are numerous lipid-laden macrophages subjacent to necrotic fat cells.

Treatment No other active management required.

Discussion Fat necrosis of the breast is a unilateral localized process associated with **trauma**, breast biopsy, reduction mammoplasty, and radiation. It is easily confused with cancer due to induration, fibrosis, dystrophic calcification, and retraction of overlying skin; the key distinction is the **presence of pain**.

ID/CC	A 32-year-old woman presents with **painful bilateral breast masses**.
HPI	The **pain is cyclic** in nature and **increases in her premenstrual phase**, at which time the **masses enlarge rapidly and then shrink**. She feels that both breasts are nodular and is concerned that she may have cancer.
PE	Mildly tender mass palpable in upper and outer quadrant of right and left breast; both **breasts nodular with multiple thickened areas**; no changes in overlying skin or nipple noted (vs. breast cancer); no axillary lymphadenopathy found.
Labs	Aspiration from breast mass reveals nonbloody fluid; **mass disappears completely after aspiration**.
Imaging	Mammo: nodularity and benign calcifications, no malignant features.
Gross Pathology	Cysts of various sizes ranging from microscopic to several millimeters surrounded by dense fibrotic tissue; contains clear or brown fluid.
Micro Pathology	Proliferation of acini in lobules (SCLEROSING ADENOSIS).
Treatment	Reassurance and symptomatic management.
Discussion	Fibrocystic disease of the breast is common in women between the ages of 35 and 55 and carries an increased risk of invasive breast cancer in patients with epithelial hyperplasia and atypia. Fibrocystic changes may result from hormone imbalances with either an excess of estrogen or a deficiency of progesterone.

ID/CC   A 59-year-old white female comes to her family doctor because of a presumed "infection" in her right **breast**; she complains of **pain and swelling**.

HPI   Her history is unremarkable.

PE   VS: **no fever** or other systemic sign of infection. PE: right breast warm, **rock-hard, and swollen with no areas of fluctuation; one-third of breast erythematous** with shiny overlying skin having **peau d'orange** appearance; **painful** to touch and pressure; several axillary **lymph nodes enlarged** and **firm**; some **coalescent**.

Labs   Routine lab work normal.

Micro Pathology   Large spheroidal cells and fine stroma infiltrated by lymphocytes on breast skin biopsy; lymphatic blood vessels occluded by tumor cells.

Treatment   Chemotherapy and radiotherapy, hormone therapy; poor prognosis.

Discussion   Inflammatory carcinoma of the breast is defined as breast cancer with angiolymphatic spread; it is characterized by a malignant course with early and widespread metastases. Perform skin biopsy in patients diagnosed with breast infection who do not respond promptly to antibiotic treatment.

Atlas Link   UCV1 PM-P3-039

ID/CC	A **35-year-old** female rushes to the emergency room and waits to see a doctor because she is concerned about a **bloody nipple discharge** that she discovered this morning.
HPI	She exercises, is very health conscious, and always has safe sex.
PE	Palpation around left nipple reveals **blood coming from one of the duct openings** and a **small, soft lump** beneath areola; no breast masses or axillary lymphadenopathy.
Imaging	Mammo: negative. Ductography: dilated duct with intraluminal filling defect.
Gross Pathology	Epithelial papillary growth with fibrotic components, characteristically located **within a lactiferous duct**.
Micro Pathology	No cellular atypia or anaplastic changes on specimen of bloody discharge; only blood intermixed with foamy macrophages and benign ductal epithelium with fibrovascular core.
Treatment	Surgical resection of lactiferous duct.
Discussion	Papilloma of the breast is a benign proliferation of ductal epithelial tissue and is the most common cause of serous/sanguineous discharge.

ID/CC A 46-year-old **woman** presents with a palpable mass in the left breast.

HPI The patient has been admitted to the hospital to obtain an excisional biopsy and for planning further management. The **patient's older sister recently died of metastatic breast cancer**.

PE Left breast mass on palpation; nipples normally located without evidence of retraction; no evidence of axillary lymphadenopathy or hepatomegaly.

Imaging Mammo: frequently normal or an asymmetric density without definable margins.

Gross Pathology Firm, white, irregularly shaped 3-cm mass was removed from each breast.

Micro Pathology Histologic sections reveal terminal lobules distended by intermediate-sized cells with scant mitotic activity; neoplastic cells infiltrate the stroma with individual neoplastic cells in a single file (INDIAN FILE PATTERN) that surrounds the terminal lobule in a target-appearing fashion.

Treatment Modified radical mastectomy with axillary lymph node sampling; radiotherapy; adjuvant chemotherapy if required. Frequent mammographic surveillance is needed owing to the **high incidence of a second primary in the same or opposite breast**.

Discussion Infiltrating lobular carcinoma is the most common malignancy of the terminal lobule. It accounts for 10% to 13% of all breast cancers.

Atlas Link `UCVII` PM-P3-041

ID/CC	A 68-year-old white woman visits her dermatologist because of a long-standing **itching, painless, scaling, and oozing erythematous rash** over her right **nipple**.
HPI	Her **first menstrual period** started at **age 9**, and she has **never** been married or **had children**; her **menopause started at age 56**.
PE	**Nipple** on right breast **retracted** and appears **eczematous** with **redness**, some edema, and **desquamation; oozing** of yellowish exudate; painless left axillary **lymphadenopathy**; no hepatomegaly or lumps in opposite breast.
Gross Pathology	Ductal carcinoma with extension to overlying skin.
Micro Pathology	Characteristic cells are scattered in the epidermis and are mucin positive and have large nuclei and abundant, pale-staining cytoplasm (PAGET'S CELLS).
Treatment	Modified radical mastectomy with axillary lymph node dissection and tamoxifen therapy.
Discussion	Paget's carcinoma is a scaly skin lesion in the **areola and nipple** arising from **ductal adenocarcinoma** within subareolar excretory ducts and progressing outward.
Atlas Link	UCV1 PG-P3-042

ID/CC A **52-year-old** unmarried white **nulliparous female** smoker with **early menarche** presents with a **painless lump** in her right breast.

HPI The patient has a **history of atypical hyperplasia** of the right breast. Her **mother died of breast cancer** at 46 years of age.

PE A 3-cm, **fixed, hard, and nontender mass** in **upper outer quadrant** of right breast; **retraction of overlying skin and nipple**; no nipple discharge; **palpable axillary lymph nodes** on right side.

Labs Routine lab work normal; normal alkaline phosphatase (no bone metastases).

Imaging Mammo: **spiculated mass with architectural distortion and multiple clustered pleomorphic microcalcifications**; skin thickening and retraction. CXR: no evidence of metastasis.

Gross Pathology Hard, irregular whitish mass with granules of calcification and focal yellow areas of necrosis. Profound **fibrosis with induration** in stroma (DESMOPLASTIC REACTION).

Micro Pathology FNA: large pleomorphic cells arranged in glands, cords, nests, and sheets in dense fibrous stroma; tumor cells **estrogen and progesterone receptor negative** by flow cytometry. Core biopsy: anaplastic cells with high mitotic index consistent with infiltrating ductal adenocarcinoma, not otherwise specified.

Treatment Surgery; tamoxifen (for estrogen-receptor-positive tumors in premenopausal women); adjuvant chemotherapy with possible bone marrow transplantation; radiotherapy.

Discussion Infiltrating ductal breast carcinoma is the **most common type of breast cancer**. Approximately one in nine women in the United States will develop breast cancer. Risk factors include **family history, early menarche, late menopause, obesity, exogenous estrogens, atypical hyperplasia of breast, and breast cancer in the opposite breast**.

Atlas Link UCV1 PM-P3-043

ID/CC	A **25-year-old** black female visits her family doctor for a **painless right breast lump** that she discovered on self-examination; she is otherwise asymptomatic.
HPI	Her medical history is unremarkable.
PE	**Small, encapsulated, well-defined, rubbery, freely movable** 3-cm mass in right lower quadrant of right breast; no overlying skin changes; no nipple retraction; no lymphadenopathy; other breast normal.
Labs	All routine lab work normal.
Imaging	Mammo: oval low-density lesion with smooth margins; **"popcorn calcifications"** seen with degeneration.
Gross Pathology	Solid mass; no areas of necrosis or hemorrhage (central myxoid degeneration in older patients).
Micro Pathology	Glandular structures with ductal and stromal proliferation with no cellular atypia.
Treatment	Surgical excision.
Discussion	Fibroadenoma is the **most common benign breast tumor in young women**; it sometimes enlarges during pregnancy or normal menstrual cycles.
Atlas Link	U C V 1 PM-P3-044

ID/CC	A 22-year-old **female** presents with an **abnormal cervical Pap smear**.
HPI	She has no history of irregular menstrual bleeding, postcoital bleeding, intermenstrual bleeding, or vaginal discharge. She delivered her **first baby at the age of 18** and has had **multiple sexual partners**.
Imaging	Colposcopy reveals a suspicious area from which a biopsy is taken.
Micro Pathology	Biopsy shows loss of normal orientation of squamous cells; atypical cells seen with wrinkled nuclei and perinuclear halos involving full thickness of squamous epithelium; basement membrane intact.
Treatment	Cone biopsy of area with regular follow-up examinations.
Discussion	Cervical dysplasia is a precursor of cervical squamous cell carcinoma; it is associated with **infection with human papillomavirus (HPV) types 16, 18, and 31**.
Atlas Link	UCV1 PM-P3-045

CERVICAL CARCINOMA (IN SITU)

ID/CC	A 29-year-old **Vietnamese female** visits her family doctor because of protracted **nausea, vaginal bleeding, dyspnea, and hemoptysis**.
HPI	Her history reveals one previous normal gestation and one spontaneous abortion as well as a dilatation and curettage 4 months ago for a **hydatidiform mole**.
PE	Vaginal examination with speculum reveals **bluish-red vascular tumor** and **enlarged uterus;** adnexa and ovaries normal.
Labs	**Markedly elevated** serum and urinary **hCG levels**.
Imaging	CXR: **multiple metastatic nodules** ("CANNONBALL" SECONDARY LESIONS).
Micro Pathology	Exaggerated trophoblastic (cytotrophoblastic and syncytiotrophoblastic) tissue proliferation with endometrial penetration; cellular atypia and hematogenous/lymphatic spread.
Treatment	Chemotherapy; follow-up with serial serum hCG levels.
Discussion	Choriocarcinoma is a malignant gestational tumor that may develop during normal pregnancy, after evacuation of hydatidiform mole, or after previous spontaneous abortions.
Atlas Link	⬚C⬚ **PM-P3-046**

ID/CC	A 33-year-old Hispanic **multigravida** in her 20th week of pregnancy comes to the gynecologist's office complaining of a **mass in her abdomen**.
HPI	She is **pregnant for the fifth time**. She has had no prior abortions or C-sections.
PE	VS: BP normal. PE: no edema; uterus correct height for gestational age (at level of umbilicus); **ill-defined, painless, nonmovable mass** 5 cm from midline on mesogastrium; skin not red or warm; no exudate; no fluctuation; **mass seems to disappear on contraction of rectus muscle**.
Labs	Routine lab work on blood, urine, and stool normal.
Imaging	CT/MR, abdomen: circumscribed mass.
Gross Pathology	Coarsely trabeculated tumor resembling scar tissue; appears to **arise from musculoaponeurotic wall**.
Micro Pathology	Elongated, spindle-shaped cells; fibroblastic process; no evidence of atypical mitoses on biopsy.
Treatment	Surgical excision; radiotherapy.
Discussion	A type of fibromatosis of the anterior abdominal wall in women, desmoid tumor is associated with previous trauma, multiple pregnancies, and Gardner's syndrome. It **frequently recurs after excision**.

ID/CC A 16-year-old girl is seen with complaints of **colicky lower abdominal pain** together with nausea and vomiting associated with the **onset of menses**.

HPI She achieved menarche at 14, and her initial cycles were irregular but painless (due to anovulation). She does not complain of any irregularity or excessive bleeding and has no urinary complaints or diarrhea.

PE Abdominal exam normal; gynecologic exam reveals blood-stained pad; pelvic exam not performed due to intact hymen; rectal exam normal.

Labs Routine lab parameters normal.

Treatment Symptomatic relief with **prostaglandin synthetase inhibitors** such as mefenamic acid or naproxen sodium; intractable symptoms may require **suppression of ovulation** using combined estrogen/progesterone or progestogens.

Discussion **Primary dysmenorrhea** is defined as **painful periods** for which no organic or psychological cause can be found; the pain is colicky and usually begins shortly after or at the onset of menses. It is thought to be due to an increase in the production of prostaglandins, leading to uterine vasoconstriction and painful contractions. Occurring **only during ovulatory cycles**, primary dysmenorrhea is most commonly found in women under the age of 20.

ID/CC	A 60-year-old **obese, nulliparous** white **female** presents with intermittent **postmenopausal vaginal bleeding** of 3 months' duration.
HPI	She has a history of **diabetes, hypertension**, and **infertility with polycystic ovaries; menopause began at 56 years of age**.
PE	**Uterus is not enlarged** on bimanual palpation.
Labs	CBC: mild anemia. Stool and urine tests within normal limits.
Imaging	US, pelvis: **thickening** of **endometrial stripe**.
Gross Pathology	Hysteroscopic biopsy performed with dilatation and curettage; **fungating mass** visualized.
Micro Pathology	**Adenocarcinoma**.
Treatment	Radiation therapy; hysterectomy.
Discussion	Endometrial carcinoma is an **estrogen-dependent** cancer and is an important differential diagnosis of postmenopausal bleeding.

ENDOMETRIAL CARCINOMA

ID/CC	A 27-year-old white female is admitted to the **infertility clinic** for evaluation of her **inability to conceive**; she also complains of **pain during intercourse** (DYSPAREUNIA) and **pain during menses** (DYSMENORRHEA).
HPI	She is **nulligravida**. She admits to having **rectal pain during menstruation**; she also complains of having an **abundant menstrual period** (MENORRHAGIA OR HYPERMENORRHEA).
PE	**Bluish spots in posterior fornix** on vaginal speculum exam; on bimanual exam, **fixed, tender bilateral ovarian masses palpable** during menstruation; **induration in pouch of Douglas** with **multiple small nodules** palpable through posterior fornix.
Imaging	Laparoscopy, pelvis: ovaries adhere to broad ligament and show retraction and scarring in addition to **endometriomas**, with dense peritubal and periovarian **adhesions** and **thickening of uterosacral ligaments**. US, pelvis: nonspecific cystic enlargement of ovaries.
Gross Pathology	Brownish nodules on uterosacral ligaments, ovaries, and pouch of Douglas.
Micro Pathology	Laparoscopic biopsy of affected areas shows nodules to consist of otherwise normal-looking, functioning endometrial glands.
Treatment	Oral contraceptives, progestogens, danazol, GnRH, surgical removal/coagulation of lesions.
Discussion	Endometriosis refers to endometrial tissue that is present outside the uterus and produces symptoms that vary with location. Endometrial implants (endometriomas or **"chocolate cysts"**) most frequently involve both **ovaries**.
Atlas Link	UCV1 PM-P3-050

ID/CC	A 25-year-old Filipina in her **20th week of pregnancy** presents with **vaginal bleeding but no pain**.
HPI	She has been feeling inordinately **nauseated** and has suffered from ringing in her ears.
PE	VS: moderate hypertension (BP 150/95). **Uterus large for gestational age** (three finger breadths above umbilicus); lower extremity 2+ **nonpitting edema**.
Labs	**Markedly increased β-hCG**. UA: **proteinuria** but no casts seen on microscopic exam. Elevated blood uric acid level. Karyotype: diploid XX (complete mole); triploid XXY or XXX (partial mole).
Imaging	US, pelvis: complex **"snowstorm" appearance** and **no fetal parts** in uterine cavity.
Gross Pathology	Characteristic appearance of **clusters of grapes**.
Micro Pathology	Chorionic villi markedly enlarged and hydropic with surrounding cyto- and syncytiotrophoblastic tissue proliferation and lack of adequate vascular supply.
Treatment	Dilatation and suction curettage, periodic determination of hCG levels to identify development of invasive mole or choriocarcinoma.
Discussion	A gestational neoplasm that may present as painless vaginal bleeding, **preeciampsia** in the first trimester, or **hyperemesis** gravidarum, hydatidiform mole may develop into **malignant choriocarcinoma** (20%).

ID/CC	A **53-year-old female** complains of **increasing fatigue, insomnia, and depression**.
HPI	For the past 6 months she has had episodes in which her **face and neck have become hot and red** (HOT FLASHES). She has been **amenorrheic for the past 7 months**; prior to this, her menstrual history was normal.
PE	**Thinning of the skin; hirsutism; atrophic vaginal mucosa** with decreased secretions.
Labs	**Increased 24-hour urinary gonadotropins** (LH and FSH).
Imaging	XR, plain: **osteoporosis** of thoracolumbar spine.
Treatment	**Estrogen replacement therapy** beneficial.
Discussion	The estrogen deficiency state produced by menopause has short-range (hot flashes), medium-range (vaginal atrophy), and long-range (osteoporosis) consequences that can be relieved or prevented by estrogen replacement. Common side effects in patients taking hormone replacement therapy include irregular bleeding, weight gain, fluid retention, and endometrial hyperplasia. Nevertheless, postmenopausal bleeding should be worked up with an endometrial biopsy to rule out endometrial cancer.

ID/CC   A **56-year-old white nulliparous woman** is referred for evaluation of a **pelvic mass** found on a routine physical.

HPI   She reports **increased frequency of micturition** and **irregular periods** until they ceased 3 years ago. **She has a history of breast cancer in the distant past**.

PE   **Large cystic mass** the size of a grapefruit in right pelvis that can be felt above the pubis symphysis.

Labs   **CA-125 levels elevated**; LFTs normal.

Imaging   CT/US, pelvis: **cystic pelvic mass arising out of right ovary**.

Gross Pathology   Partly solid and partly cystic mass.

Micro Pathology   Papillary structures of neoplastic ciliated columnar cells; **psammoma bodies**.

Treatment   Surgical staging and resection; chemotherapy.

Discussion   Ovarian cancer is the third most common type of gynecologic cancer; the **serous type** is **most common** and is **often bilateral**. It is often advanced at the time of diagnosis (omental masses, liver masses, ascites).

ID/CC	A 20-year-old Asian **female** visits her family doctor because of **chronic, intermittent left lower quadrant pain**.
HPI	The pain is not accompanied by dyspareunia, menstrual irregularity, vaginal discharge, abdominal distention, nausea, vomiting, or diarrhea. It is not correlated with her menstrual periods.
PE	**Left adnexal mass** on bimanual exam; uterosacral ligaments normal; pouch of Douglas normal; McBurney's point nontender; no evidence of ascites.
Labs	Routine lab work on blood, urine, and stool normal; CA-125 levels not elevated.
Imaging	US, pelvis: **large (5-cm) simple cyst in left ovary**.
Micro Pathology	Vaginal smears for cytohormonal evaluation reveal excessive estrogenic stimulation and lack of progestational effect.
Treatment	Follow-up by ultrasound (sizable percentage disappear spontaneously); laparoscopic removal if persistent.
Discussion	Follicular ovarian cyst is the most common cause of ovarian enlargement.

OVARIAN CYST—FOLLICULAR

ID/CC	A **25-year-old woman** complains of **loss of weight** and intense right lower abdominal pain and nausea that began when she went jogging yesterday afternoon.
HPI	Intermittent episodes of similar pain have occurred over the past several days. She has regular menstrual cycles with average flow and no dysmenorrhea and had her last period 3 weeks ago.
PE	VS: mild hypotension; normal HR (HR 90). PE: **right lower quadrant tenderness**; pelvic exam reveals tender, mobile 6-cm **right adnexal mass** anterior to uterus.
Labs	CBC: normal; pregnancy test negative.
Imaging	XR, KUB: irregular **calcified** mass in region of right ovary. US, pelvis: **cystic tumor** about 8 cm in diameter replacing the right ovary.
Gross Pathology	Cystic mass replacing the right ovary; thin, **fibrous wall with solid nodule at one aspect containing sebaceous material and matted hair**; tooth structures also seen.
Micro Pathology	Mature tissue elements **representing all three germ cell layers** are present, including skin with adnexal structures, bone, cartilage, teeth, thyroid, bronchi, intestine, and neural tissue.
Treatment	Surgical resection curative.
Discussion	Primary benign teratomas or dermoid cysts originate from germ cells; tumors are cystic and contain elements of all three germ cell layers. Complications of teratomas include torsion, infection, rupture leading to chemical peritonitis, infertility, secretion of thyroid hormone leading to hyperthyroidism (STRUMA OVARII), and carcinoid syndrome due to serotonin secretion; rarely, squamous cell carcinoma may develop in a dermoid cyst.
Atlas Link	UCV1 PG-P3-055

OVARIAN TERATOMA

ID/CC A **23-year-old** married **woman** is seen with complaints of **inability to conceive** after a year of unprotected intercourse (INFERTILITY).

HPI Her last menstrual period was 3 months ago, and since menarche she **has only 4 to 5 periods each year** (OLIGOMENORRHEA); a pregnancy test at home was negative. She also complains of **excessive facial hair**. Her **father was diabetic**.

PE Patient **obese**; excessive **facial hair and male-pattern hair distribution on rest of body** (HIRSUTISM) but no virilization; pelvic exam normal; secondary sexual characteristics well developed.

Labs Elevated **LH; decreased FSH** and loss of normal periodicity (LH > FSH, 3:1 ratio); **serum testosterone and androstenedione elevated; serum estradiol** (total and free) within normal limits in early and midfollicular phases; **pattern of secretion abnormal with no preovulatory or midluteal increase**; TSH and prolactin levels normal.

Imaging US, transvaginal (high resolution): morphologic features of **polycystic ovaries** (multiple peripheral follicles < 8 mm in diameter; prominent echodense stroma).

Gross Pathology Ovaries enlarged with **pearly-white capsule** and multiple cysts averaging 1 cm in diameter within stroma.

Micro Pathology Cysts **lined by granulosa and theca cells**, the latter luteinized; stroma shows **hyperthecosis** and fibrosis.

Treatment Reduce weight; ovulation induction with clomiphene; laparoscopic ovarian diathermy or laser drilling in drug-resistant cases; low-dose combined contraceptive pill if contraception is desired.

Discussion Polycystic ovarian syndrome (**Stein–Leventhal syndrome**) is a clinical syndrome of **obesity, hirsutism, and secondary amenorrhea or oligomenorrhea with infertility due to anovulation**, accompanied by multiple-follicle cysts within both ovaries. PCOS patients are at increased risk for breast and endometrial carcinomas (due to unopposed LH stimulation).

Atlas Link UCV1 PG-P3-056

ID/CC   A 17-year-old white **female** visits her family physician because she **has never had a menstrual period** (PRIMARY AMENORRHEA) and **lacks breast development**.

HPI   She has a history of **low birth weight** and lymphedema.

PE   **Short stature**; low-set ears; **webbed neck**; cubitus valgus; low hairline; **shield-like chest with widely spaced nipples; harsh systolic murmur heard on back** (due to coarctation of aorta); hypoplastic nails; short fourth metacarpals; high-arched palate; **absence of pubic and axillary hair**; small clitoris and uterus; ovaries not palpable.

Labs   High serum and urine FSH and LH; **no Barr bodies** on buccal smear. Karyotype: **45,XO**.

Imaging   US, pelvis: infantile streak ovaries. Echo: bicuspid aortic valve.

Gross Pathology   Fibrotic and atrophic ovaries.

Micro Pathology   Absence of follicles in ovaries; normal ovarian stroma replaced by **fibrous streaks**.

Treatment   Growth hormone and androgens for increase in stature; subsequent estrogen therapy to protect against osteoporosis.

Discussion   The most common karyotype is 45,XO; less commonly, mosaicism. Turner's syndrome is associated with frequent skeletal, renal (horseshoe kidney), and cardiovascular anomalies.

ID/CC	A 39-year-old **black female** presents with a several-month-long history of **profuse menstruation** (HYPERMENORRHEA) **and frequent menstrual periods** (POLYMENORRHEA).
HPI	Further questioning also reveals **painful periods** (DYSMENORRHEA) and increasing **urinary frequency**. She has a history of **infertility** and **recurrent spontaneous abortions**.
PE	**Enlarged, irregular uterus** on bimanual palpation with several masses on posterior wall.
Labs	CBC/PBS: hypochromic, microcytic anemia.
Imaging	US, pelvis: **multiple heterogeneous masses** distorting uterus.
Gross Pathology	Occur in myometrium (95% are intramural) and are round, firm, and well circumscribed.
Micro Pathology	Interlacing bundles of uniform, differentiated, elongated smooth muscle cells with few mitoses and no anaplasia; malignant transformation rare.
Treatment	Myomectomy; hysterectomy.
Discussion	The **most common tumor of the uterus** and the **most common tumor in women**, uterine fibroids are **estrogen-dependent** and commonly occur after 30 years of age; they tend to regress after menopause.
Atlas Link	UCV1 PG-P3-058

UTERINE FIBROIDS

ID/CC A 60-year-old woman visits her gynecologist because of a **foul-smelling, blood-tinged, purulent vaginal discharge**.

HPI She has never been married and **has never been pregnant**. She is hypertensive and takes oral hypoglycemic agents for diabetes mellitus.

PE VS: BP normal at present. PE: overweight; **fleshy, bulky, fungating tumor** protruding from cervical os on vaginal speculum exam.

Imaging CT/MR: large, complex mass arising from uterus.

Gross Pathology Large, fleshy tumor of myometrium with areas of necrosis and hemorrhage.

Micro Pathology Background of spindle-shaped cells with **more than 10 mitoses per high-power field** on biopsy; many mitoses have abnormal mitotic spindle.

Treatment Adriamycin, progestins, combination chemotherapy.

Discussion A highly aggressive malignant tumor of myometrium, leiomyosarcoma of the uterus may arise in a leiomyoma or de novo. It spreads by contiguity, hematogenously, and through lymphatics.

Atlas Link UCV1 PG-P3-059

ID/CC   A **65-year-old woman** is referred for intractable vulvar growth and **pruritus**.

HPI   She has also felt an obstruction in the flow of her urine. She was a **prostitute** and was treated often for STDs. She is a **chronic smoker**.

PE   Gynecologic exam reveals excoriation marks over vulva; exophytic growth arising from left labia majora; left inguinal lymphadenopathy.

Labs   Cystoscopy reveals lower urethral stenosis (due to involvement by vulvar growth).

Gross Pathology   Gross examination reveals firm, exophytic growth.

Micro Pathology   Microscopic exam of punch biopsy specimen reveals invasive, well-differentiated **squamous cell carcinoma with keratinization**.

Treatment   Confirm diagnosis; preoperative radiotherapy to shrink tumor mass; radical vulvectomy with lymph node dissection.

Discussion   Vulvar cancer is a disease of **older women** with a mean age of 60 years. It is associated with **smoking**, and its recent increase in incidence among younger women is associated with **papillomavirus**. Carcinoma in situ (vulvar intraepithelial neoplasia, or VIN) and squamous dysplasia are considered precursor lesions.

ID/CC   A 75-year-old white **woman** visits her gynecologist for a routine checkup and is found to have **white spots** on her **genitalia**.

HPI   She complains of slight outer vaginal **itching** but denies any postmenopausal bleeding, vaginal discharge, or drug intake.

PE   **Hypochromic macules** on labia majora extending to perineum and inner thighs in patchy distribution with **scale formation** (DESQUAMATION); **skin thickened and rough** (HYPERKERATOTIC); no regional lymphadenopathy; atrophic vaginitis on vaginal speculum exam.

Micro Pathology   Biopsy reveals hyperkeratosis and fibrosis with thinning of squamous epithelium; lymphocytic inflammatory infiltration, most prevalent surrounding blood vessels; no chronic inflammatory response; no signs of malignant transformation.

Treatment   **Biopsy**; subsequent treatment dependent on diagnosis.

Discussion   **Vulvar leukoplakia** is a clinical diagnosis that can be attributed to a variety of disorders that all produce white patches. Causes may be benign disorders such as vitiligo, as well as inflammatory conditions, premalignant conditions (e.g., dystrophies), or squamous cell carcinoma. **Always perform a biopsy.**

ID/CC	A **73-year-old** woman is brought to a gynecologist by her daughter, who became aware of a **genital ulcer** while helping her mother shower.
HPI	Her history reveals **weight loss** and **dyspnea** together with hypertension and arthritis.
PE	Hard, nodular, 5-mm **pigmented and ulcerated** lesion on upper left **labia minora**; no inguinal lymphadenopathy; scattered crepitant rales on chest auscultation.
Labs	CBC/PBS: slight anemia.
Imaging	CXR: **multiple metastatic nodules**.
Micro Pathology	Biopsy reveals malignant melanoma cells with lymphocytic reaction infiltrating into underlying dermis; cells stain **positive for S100 antigen** and are **negative for mucin**.
Treatment	Surgery with regional lymph node dissection and adjuvant chemotherapy.
Discussion	Vulvar malignant melanoma is the second most common vulvar malignancy (the first is squamous cell carcinoma); metastasis and prognosis depend on the extent of vertical growth.

ID/CC	A 25-year-old **woman** presents with **amenorrhea** of 6 weeks' duration and **pelvic pain** over the past day.
HPI	She has a history of **vaginal spotting off and on** for the past 2 weeks and has been using an **IUD** for the past 3 years. She has no history of vaginal discharge and no urinary symptoms, and her previous menstrual history is normal. She has had multiple bouts of **pelvic inflammatory disease**.
PE	VS: BP normal. PE: pallor; abdominal distention and decreased bowel sounds; **cervical motion tenderness**; uterus soft and slightly enlarged on pelvic exam; **soft, tender, boggy mass in right adnexa and pouch of Douglas**.
Labs	CBC: anemia. **hCG levels lower than expected** for this period of gestation; culdocentesis reveals presence of blood in cul-de-sac.
Imaging	US, pelvis: **no products of conception in uterine cavity**; doughnut-shaped mass in right adnexa; echogenic free fluid in cul-de-sac.
Gross Pathology	Extrauterine pregnancy, most commonly tubal.
Micro Pathology	Uterine curettage reveals presence of Arias–Stella reaction in the **absence of villi**.
Treatment	Laparoscopic linear salpingostomy and segmental resection; methotrexate.
Discussion	Other risk factors for ectopic pregnancy include **previous tubal surgery**, tubal ligation, **endometriosis, previous ectopic pregnancy**, and ovulation induction.

ID/CC	A 38-year-old **grand multipara** develops a marked drop in her blood pressure following **uncontrolled bleeding immediately after delivery**.
HPI	She delivered **twins** at 35 weeks' gestation with **polyhydramnios**.
PE	VS: **hypotension; tachycardia**. PE: anxious; pallor; low central venous pressure; **uterus soft and flabby** with indistinct outline.
Labs	CBC: anemia; mildly decreased hematocrit. Coagulation profile normal.
Gross Pathology	Uterus **grossly overdistended and flabby**.
Treatment	**Fluid resuscitation; blood transfusion; uterine massage**; maintain contraction with an oxytocin infusion; ergotamine for vasoconstriction; if found, **remove retained placenta**; check for cervical, vaginal, or uterine lacerations and uterine rupture; hypogastric artery ligation and/or hysterectomy if other measures fail.
Discussion	Primary postpartum hemorrhage (PPH) is defined as loss of 500 mL or more of blood within 24 hours of a vaginal delivery (1,000 mL after a C-section) or any amount of bleeding that is sufficient to produce a hemodynamic compromise; primary causes include uterine atony, retained placenta, and soft tissue injury. Factors associated with an increased risk of uterine atony and retained placenta include **high multiparity, a maternal age greater than 35 years, delivery after an antepartum hemorrhage, multiple pregnancies, polyhydramnios, a past history of PPH, and coagulation disorders**. Sheehan's syndrome—a clinical syndrome of hypopituitarism secondary to ischemic pituitary necrosis—is a peculiar complication of massive postpartum hemorrhage.

ID/CC	A 28-year-old **woman** presents with **swelling of her entire left leg** of 1 day's duration.
HPI	She delivered a normal full-term male baby 2 days ago.
PE	Left leg **erythematous, warm, swollen**, and **tender**.
Labs	Routine tests normal; normal clotting profile.
Imaging	US, Doppler: clot in left femoral vein. Venography: confirmatory "gold standard" but usually not required.
Treatment	IV heparin and monitoring of clotting time and PTT; elevation of limb; analgesics and soaks.
Discussion	**Phlegmasia alba dolens** (painful white leg) is due to iliofemoral vein thrombosis occurring in late pregnancy and **postpartum**; it is related to **compression by a gravid uterus** and **hypercoagulability** of pregnancy.

ID/CC	A 30-year-old **woman** presents with fatigue, **significant weight loss**, and **amenorrhea** of 2 years' duration.
HPI	She had a baby 2 years ago and suffered **significant postpartum bleeding**. She bottle-fed her baby because she was **unable to lactate** after delivery.
PE	VS: **hypotension** (BP 85/60). PE: skin tenting; fine wrinkling around eyes and mouth; loss of axillary and pubic hair.
Labs	**Decreased levels of trophic hormones (FSH, LH, ACTH, TSH, GH, prolactin)**; decreased levels of target gland hormones (T_3, T_4, cortisol, estrogens).
Imaging	MR, pituitary (usually before and after injection of gadolinium DTPA): abnormal signal in pituitary gland.
Gross Pathology	Soft, pale, and hemorrhagic pituitary gland in early stages; shrunken, fibrous, and firm in later stages.
Treatment	Hormone replacement: cortisol; levothyroxine (T_4); estrogen-progesterone replacement.
Discussion	Sheehan's syndrome is most commonly caused by **postpartum infarction of the pituitary**. During pregnancy, the anterior pituitary grows to nearly twice its normal size. During delivery, loss of blood or hypovolemia decreases flow to the pituitary, inducing vasospasm that leads to **ischemic necrosis** of the anterior pituitary. The posterior pituitary is supplied by arteries and is therefore much less susceptible to ischemia. Loss of trophic hormones leads to atrophy of target organs. Ischemic necrosis may also occur in males and in nonpregnant females (trauma, sickle cell anemia, disseminated intravascular coagulation, vascular accidents).

SHEEHAN'S SYNDROME

ID/CC	A 30-year-old white **primigravida** at **36 weeks of gestation** visits her obstetrician for the first time in her pregnancy complaining of **swollen legs and headache**.
HPI	Her medical history is unremarkable, and her pregnancy had apparently developed with no complications until the onset of her symptoms.
PE	VS: **hypertension** (BP 170/110). PE: **excessive weight gain** (19 kg); funduscopic exam does not show changes of hypertensive retinopathy; 3+ **pitting pedal edema**; 1+ periorbital edema; fundal height appropriate; fetal parts palpable; fetal heart sounds normal.
Labs	CBC/PBS: complete blood counts and coagulation profile normal. Serum uric acid concentrations raised; mildly elevated AST and ALT; 3+ **proteinuria**.
Imaging	US, OB: single live fetus; lie longitudinal; presentation cephalic; normal biophysical profile; **placental infarctions** seen.
Micro Pathology	Endothelial cell swelling with obliteration of glomerular capillary lumen on renal biopsy.
Treatment	Antihypertensive agents; delivery of fetus and placenta, usually by C-section.
Discussion	Preeclampsia occurs in 5% of all pregnancies; it is most common during the **last trimester of a first pregnancy**. It is characterized by the triad of **hypertension, proteinuria, and edema**. Progression to eclampsia may occur with visual disturbances, seizures, and coma.

ID/CC	A **14-year-old male** is admitted to the hospital complaining of **pain** and **swelling** in the left **leg**.
HPI	The pain has been present for 2 months but has become progressively worse over that period. There is no history of trauma or infection.
PE	VS: **mild fever**. PE: tenderness and fusiform swelling over left femur.
Labs	Elevated ESR. Karyotype: **translocation of the long arms of chromosomes 11 and 22**.
Imaging	XR, left femur: lytic lesion in medullary zone of midshaft with cortical destruction and **"onion-skin"** appearance. CXR: no evidence of metastatic spread.
Gross Pathology	Large areas of bone lysis as tumors erode cancellous trabeculae of long bones outward to cortex.
Micro Pathology	Biopsy of bone reveals sheets of uniform, small cells resembling lymphocytes; in many places tumor cells surround a central clear area, forming a **"pseudorosette." Cell origin of tumor is unknown**.
Treatment	**"Melt" tumor with radiotherapy**; surgical resection; chemotherapy; regular follow-up for recurrence.
Discussion	**Diaphysis** of the long bones is the **most common site of occurrence** of Ewing's sarcoma. Five-year survival is 70% for locally resectable disease but only 30% for those with advanced metastasis.

ID/CC	A 45-year-old woman visits an orthopedist because of an **inability to extend her fourth and fifth fingers**.
HPI	She has a long-standing history of **alcohol abuse** and has been to the emergency room several times for alcoholic gastritis.
PE	Mild icterus; palmar erythema; muscle wasting; malnourishment; abdomen reveals 2+ ascitic fluid (due to alcoholic liver damage); **fourth and fifth fingers of right hand reveal flexion contracture** with nodular thickening and thick bands of tissue palpable upon drawing examining finger across palm.
Gross Pathology	Infiltration of palmar fascia with fibrous tissue and subsequent contraction deformity.
Micro Pathology	Infiltration of pretendinous fascia with myofibroblasts with fibrosis of pretendinous bands.
Treatment	Surgery (release of contractures and adhesions); frequently recurs.
Discussion	Also called palmar fibromatosis, Dupuytren's contracture is of unknown etiology but is associated with alcoholism and **manual labor**. It is associated with diabetes and anticonvulsant medications.

ORTHOPEDICS

ID/CC	A **60-year-old woman** is brought to the orthopedic clinic with complaints of **pain in the left hip and inability to bear weight** on the left leg.
HPI	**Three years** ago she sustained a **fracture of the neck of the femur** that was treated with internal fixation. She is an **alcoholic** and has been taking **oral steroids** for many years for a chronic skin ailment.
PE	All movements at left hip are restricted by pain; unable to bear weight on the limb.
Imaging	XR, left hip: **increase in bone density of femoral head** and collapse of articular surface; dynamic hip screw in place. MR, hip: more sensitive.
Treatment	**Total hip replacement arthroplasty** significantly reduces morbidity.
Discussion	**Fracture of the neck of the femur is the most common cause** of avascular necrosis of the femoral head; other risk factors include excessive alcohol consumption, steroid therapy, radiation therapy, sickle cell anemia, and deep sea diving (**Caisson's disease**). Normally **blood is supplied to the head by three routes**: through vessels in the ligamentum teres, through capsular vessels reflected onto the femoral neck, and through branches of nutrient vessels within the substance of the bone. When the fracture occurs, nutrient vessels are necessarily severed, capsular vessels are injured to varying degrees, and **blood supply is maintained only through the vessels in the ligamentum teres**. This is a variable quantity and is often insufficient, resulting in avascular necrosis of the femoral head.

ID/CC	A **12-year-old obese male** is brought to the hospital with complaints of sudden-onset pain of the left hip along with a limp.
HPI	The pain is felt in the left groin and often radiates to the left thigh and knee.
PE	Left leg **externally rotated and about 2 cm shorter**; limited range of abduction and internal rotation; **upon flexing left hip, knee is drawn toward left axilla**.
Imaging	XR, left hip (AP view): **growth plate widened and irregular**.
Treatment	Head was fixed with pins or screws to prevent further slipping.
Discussion	Slipped femoral epiphyses affects youth **10 to 18 years old**, with boys more commonly affected than girls; affected children may be overweight and in some cases have delayed sexual development. Represents a Salter-Harris type I epiphyseal injury. Twenty-five percent are bilateral, of which 15% to 20% occur simultaneously. **Avascular necrosis** of the femoral head and **osteoarthritis** may arise as complications.

ID/CC	A 25-year-old female **athlete** is brought to the ER after she hurt her right knee.
HPI	She had **fallen on a hyperextended right knee** that has been unstable since the fall. She recalls having heard a "popping" sound at the time of the injury.
PE	Right knee exhibits effusion and **positive anterior "draw sign"** (tibia can be pulled forward on femur with knee flexed); instability of right knee joint (demonstrated by moving upper end of tibia forward on femur with knee flexed only 10 to 20 degrees [LACHMAN TEST]).
Imaging	MR, knee: indistinct, heterogenous signal in expected region of the anterior cruciate ligament.
Treatment	Surgical reconstruction; plaster cylinder for 3 weeks followed by hamstring and quadriceps exercises.
Discussion	The anterior cruciate ligament is torn by a force driving the upper end of the tibia forward relative to the femur or by hyperextension of the knee; the **posterior cruciate ligament is torn by a force driving the upper end of the tibia backward.**

ID/CC	A **60-year-old obese female** is seen with complaints of gradually progressing **stiffness and pain after use of the right knee**.
HPI	The pain and stiffness are accompanied by swelling and deformity of the joint. She also reports difficulty walking and limitation of movement.
PE	Tenderness, pain, and crepitus of right knee on motion; firm swelling (caused by underlying bony proliferations) and joint effusion; fixed deformities: bony enlargement and a varus angulation, causing limited motion at joint; hands show **bony swellings on distal interphalangeal joints** (HEBERDEN'S NODES).
Labs	Synovial fluid shows no evidence of inflammation; normal viscosity and mucin clot tests; protein, glucose, and complement levels also normal; serum rheumatoid factor not raised.
Imaging	XR, right knee (AP and lateral views): narrowing of joint space (medial > lateral); subchondral bone sclerosis; subchondral cysts and osteophytes.
Gross Pathology	Late stages of the disease show **eburnation** of joint surface, **remodeling** of joint surface, **osteophytes** around lateral margins of joint, subchondral bone cysts, and bone sclerosis.
Micro Pathology	Loss of articular cartilage, bone resorption, and irregular and variable new bone and cartilage formation.
Treatment	Pain relief, improvement of mobility, and correction of deformity; joint replacement.
Discussion	Osteoarthritis, a degenerative joint disease, is characterized by the degeneration of articular cartilage and by progressive destruction and remodeling of the joint structures. The condition affects large weight-bearing joints such as the knees, hips, and lumbar and cervical vertebrae; other joints commonly affected are the PIP, DIP, and first carpometacarpal joints. It is more common in women, and its incidence increases with age, particularly after 55.
Atlas Links	⬚CⱽＩ PG-P3-073 ⬚Cⱽ2 SUR-044

ORTHOPEDICS

ID/CC	A **12-year-old male** presents with a **swelling** above the right knee and associated pain.
HPI	There is **no history of trauma** at the site of pain. There has been **no discharge** from the swollen region and **no fever**.
PE	**Bony-hard**, tender, roughly circular swelling above right knee **(distal femur)**; overlying skin temperature normal; mechanical restriction of movement of right knee.
Labs	Normal ESR; **elevated serum alkaline phosphatase** (may be used as marker of treatment response).
Imaging	XR, plain: osteoblastic bone lesion at distal end of femur with characteristic **"sunburst" or "onion-peel"** periosteal reaction; periosteal elevation by metaphyseal tumor (CODMAN'S TRIANGLE).
Gross Pathology	Firm, whitish mass with **osteoblastic** bone sclerosis originating from **metaphysis** adjacent to epiphyseal growth plate and invading through cortex, lifting up periosteum.
Micro Pathology	Bone biopsy shows multinucleated giant cells, anaplastic cells with pleomorphism, and osteoid production with foci of sarcomatous degeneration.
Treatment	Surgical amputation; consider limb salvage; radiotherapy, chemotherapy.
Discussion	Osteogenic sarcoma is the most common primary malignant tumor of bone (excluding myeloma and lymphoma); it may be osteoblastic or osteolytic. Pathologic fractures may occur; pulmonary metastases are frequent. There is an increased risk with Paget's disease, prior radiation, and hereditary retinoblastoma.
Atlas Link	UCV1 PM-P3-074

ID/CC	A 70-year-old male immigrant from England presents with **pain** in the right leg, producing an awkward gait, along with bilateral **hearing loss**.
HPI	He has also noted a progressive **increase in his hat size**.
PE	Slight **bowing of right tibia**; normal rectal exam; mixed conductive and **sensorineural hearing loss** confirmed by audiometry; physical exam otherwise normal.
Labs	**Markedly elevated alkaline phosphatase**; mildly elevated serum calcium and phosphorus; normal serum transaminases; **increased urinary excretion of hydroxyproline**.
Imaging	XR, skull: scattered **islands of bone lysis** (OSTEOPOROSIS CIRCUMSCRIPTA); mixed **thickening** (blastic) **and lucency** (lytic lesions) of bone (COTTON-WOOL APPEARANCE). XR, leg (right side): bone soft with disorganized trabecular pattern; bowed tibia.
Gross Pathology	Expansion of bone cortex, blastic bone lesions, and bowing of long bones (thick ivory bones).
Micro Pathology	Multiple cement lines with unmineralized osteoid; indicative of excessive osteoblastic and osteoclastic activity.
Treatment	Osteotomies; calcitonin; diphosphonate; mithramycin.
Discussion	A condition of probable viral etiology, Paget's disease is characterized by osteoclastic destruction of bone initially with excessive osteoblastic repair, producing bone sclerosis. When extensive, the resulting increased blood flow leads to **high cardiac output congestive heart failure**. Other complications are **pathologic fracture and osteosarcoma** (1% of patients).

ORTHOPEDICS

PAGET'S DISEASE OF BONE

ID/CC A **5-year-old male** is brought to a physician with sudden-onset progressive severe **pain, swelling, and redness** of the right knee joint.

HPI He has had a **high-grade fever** for the past 2 days. A few days ago he **injured his right leg, and the injury subsequently became infected**; he is now unable to move his right leg properly.

PE VS: fever. PE: infected wound on right leg; right **knee red, swollen, and tender**; all movements restricted by pain.

Labs CBC: **neutrophilic leukocytosis** with shift to the left. Elevated ESR; **synovial fluid (obtained following joint aspiration) opaque and yellowish; joint effusion has WBC count > 50,000/μL**; Gram stain reveals **gram-positive cocci in clusters**; culture yields coagulase-positive *Staphylococcus aureus*.

Imaging XR, right knee: early, soft tissue swelling and joint effusion; late, articular erosions and reactive sclerosis. NUC, gallium scan: increased uptake by right knee joint.

Treatment **Broad-spectrum parenteral antibiotics** initially, then specific antibiotics following culture sensitivity reports; if necessary, joint may be opened, washed, and closed with a suction drain and immobilized until signs of inflammation subside.

Discussion Septic arthritis is caused by pyogenic organisms and is more common among children, especially males. *S. aureus* is the most common cause; other organisms include streptococci, gonococci, pneumococci, and *Neisseria meningitides*. Organisms reach the joint via hematogenous routes (most common; the primary focus may be a pyoderma, throat infection, IV drug use, etc.), secondary to adjacent osteomyelitis, or via penetrating wounds, or the condition may be iatrogenic.

Atlas Links ᵁᶜᵛ2 IM2-041A, IM2-041B

ID/CC	A 55-year-old woman presents with an **aching pain in the back of her neck**, a feeling of stiffness, and a **"grating" sensation upon movement**.
HPI	She also has a history of a vague, ill-defined, and ill-localized pain spreading over her shoulder region. She does not complain of any noticeable motor weakness or sensory loss over any part of the body and has no bladder or bowel complaints.
PE	Neck **slightly kyphotic; posterior cervical muscles tender; neck movements** slightly **restricted at extremes** due to pain; **audible crepitation on movement; diminished supinator and biceps reflex in the left upper limb**; no motor or sensory loss demonstrable.
Imaging	XR, cervical spine (lateral view): **narrowing of intervertebral disk space with formation of osteophytes at vertebral margins**, especially anteriorly.
Treatment	There is a strong tendency for the **symptoms of cervical spondylosis to subside spontaneously**. Treatment includes **analgesics, physiotherapy, and support of the neck** by a closely fitting collar of plaster or plastic. Surgical intervention is required for patients who are unresponsive to conservative therapy as well as for those with progressive myelopathy or radiculopathy.
Discussion	Degenerative arthritis occurs predominantly in the **lowest three cervical joints**. The changes **first affect the central intervertebral joints and later affect the posterior intervertebral (facet) joints. Osteophytes commonly encroach on the intervertebral foramina**, reducing the space for transmission of the cervical nerves. If the restricted space is further reduced by the traumatic edema of the contained soft tissues, manifestations of nerve pressure are likely to occur. Rarely, the spinal cord itself may suffer damage, producing a cervical myelopathy.

ORTHOPEDICS

ID/CC	A 32-year-old homeless white male is brought to the emergency room by an ambulance following **convulsions** that took place on the street.
HPI	The patient is disheveled and unshaven in his appearance. A history cannot be obtained because he is alone and unable to respond to questions.
PE	Dehydration; **jaundice; alcohol on breath**; 2-cm laceration on occipital area with no bleeding; semicomatose state with response to pain only; pupils equal; **fine tremor** in extremities; palmar erythema; **hepatomegaly**.
Labs	CBC/PBS: **macrocytic, hypochromic anemia. Elevated** direct and indirect **bilirubin; elevated AST and ALT**; AST/ALT ratio of 2:1; **elevated alkaline phosphatase; elevated PT; low serum albumin**; hypoglycemia.
Gross Pathology	**Fatty liver**; micronodular **cirrhosis**; marked **gastritis**; bronchial aspiration.
Micro Pathology	Hepatocytes distended with fat; hepatocellular necrosis; **Mallory bodies** (hyaline); cytoplasmic vacuolization of stem cells in bone marrow; myofibrillar necrosis; diffuse axonal degeneration.
Treatment	Vitamins (thiamine and folate); glucose; rehydration; treat acute withdrawal and delirium tremens (DTs) with benzodiazepines.
Discussion	Alcoholic **DTs** usually occur 2 to 5 days after cessation of drinking and are characterized by seizures, delusions, agitation, disorientation, visual and tactile hallucinations, and autonomic instability. DT prophylaxis consists of benzodiazepines and restraints to prevent damage to patient and to others. DTs have a mortality rate of 15% if untreated.

ID/CC	A **24-year-old white male** visits his family doctor complaining of **low back pain and stiffness** of the spine for almost 1 year, increasing in severity.
HPI	The back stiffness is eased by a hot shower, and worsens after prolonged inactivity.
PE	**Stooped posture**; loss of lumbar lordosis and **fixed kyphosis; tenderness over sacroiliac joints**; reduced chest expansion; prominent abdomen.
Labs	Elevated ESR; **negative rheumatoid tests; positive HLA-B27.**
Imaging	XR, plain: sclerosis and blurring of margins of **sacroiliac joints; ankylosis and fusion of vertebrae** ("BAMBOO SPINE") in long-standing cases.
Gross Pathology	Calcification of intervertebral disks and longitudinal ligaments.
Micro Pathology	Similar to rheumatoid arthritis, but in different location and no rheumatoid nodules.
Treatment	Physical therapy; NSAIDs; sulfasalazine.
Discussion	Also called Marie-Strümpell disease and associated with **HLA-B27**, this inflammatory arthritis with eventual ankylosis of the spine is typically seen in young males; long-standing cases may present with **iritis** and **aortic insufficiency**. Ankylosing spondylitis is also associated with Reiter's syndrome and inflammatory bowel disease.

ANKYLOSING SPONDYLITIS

ID/CC   A 55-year-old male is brought into the emergency department **diaphoretic** and **ashen** in appearance.

HPI   He is an experienced pilot who was on a **cross-country flight** from New York to California. His ascent was uneventful to an altitude of **30,000 feet** above mean sea level in an unpressurized airplane. After 1 hour at this cruising altitude (and while on supplemental oxygen), the pilot noticed a gradual onset of **weakness and paresthesias of the right arm**. These symptoms progressively worsened to involve both arms.

PE   VS: normal. PE: **disoriented and confused**; normal cardiac and pulmonary exam; neurologic exam revealed severe flexor weakness at the right elbow and wrist, numbness of the forearm, and impaired fine motor control.

Labs   CBC/Lytes: normal. Ventilation-perfusion scan shows no V-Q mismatch. ABGs (at room air): normal.

Imaging   CXR: mild increase in interstitial markings. Consider head CT scan if mental status changes do not improve with hyperbaric repressurization. MRI may be useful for neurologic decompression sickness (DCS) to localize area of injury.

Treatment   Initial management with **hydration, 100% oxygen delivery by mask, and transfer to a hyperbaric chamber for compression therapy**. Serious cases of DCS may require intubation and pressor agents. **Compression therapy** is the definitive treatment, and treatment should be started as soon as possible.

Discussion   **Decompression sickness**, also referred to as **Caisson's disease**, occurs when a person is subjected to a rapid reduction in ambient pressure, resulting in the formation of dissolved bubbles of nitrogen within body tissues ("the bends"). DCS can result from high-altitude exposure (i.e., an unpressurized aircraft at > 29,000 feet altitude) or from work in pressurized tunnels or caissons, and is **most commonly** associated with **compressed-air** (SCUBA) **diving**.

ID/CC	A 52-year-old white **female** complains to her family doctor of **difficulty climbing** steps for the past 6 months and difficulty washing her hair for the past 2 weeks.
HPI	She states that she does not feel tired or short of breath but that her legs and arms "just will not cooperate." She also complains of intermittent fever.
PE	**Periorbital edema** with purplish discoloration (HELIOTROPE RASH); **butterfly rash** on face and neck; Raynaud's phenomenon; **scaling of skin with redness around knuckles** (GOTTRON'S LESIONS); **proximal muscle weakness with tenderness** in all four extremities.
Labs	CBC: mild leukocytosis. **Elevated serum CK**; elevated aldolase; elevated ESR; **antinuclear antibodies (ANAs)** present, particularly against tRNA. EMG: spontaneous fibrillation.
Gross Pathology	Muscle edema progressing to muscle atrophy and fibrosis.
Micro Pathology	Muscle biopsy shows lymphocytic infiltration, primarily in a perivascular fashion but also between muscle fibers on muscle biopsy; atrophy and fibrosis seen.
Treatment	Corticosteroids; methotrexate; azathioprine.
Discussion	Dermatomyositis is an idiopathic disorder primarily affecting older females; it is frequently associated with malignancy (e.g., ovarian carcinoma).
Atlas Links	UCV2 IM2-051A, IM2-051B

RHEUMATOLOGY

ID/CC A 10-year-old male presents with a persistent **low-grade fever, skin rash, and painful swelling of both knees**.

HPI He also complains of excessive fatigue and significant anorexia. He has no history of sore throat, pedal edema/orthopnea, nocturnal dyspnea, or involuntary movements.

PE VS: fever. PE: extensive erythematous maculopapular rash; generalized lymphadenopathy; hepatosplenomegaly; arthritis of both knees; no subcutaneous nodules; no evidence of carditis; no Roth's spots on funduscopy; no petechiae over skin or mucosa; normal cardiovascular exam.

Labs CBC/PBS: leukocytosis; normocytic, normochromic anemia. Elevated ESR; blood cultures sterile; ASO titers normal; throat swab sterile; **rheumatoid factor negative**; leukocytosis with **elevated proteins and markedly low glucose and complement levels** on synovial fluid analysis. ECG: normal.

Imaging XR, knees: effusion and soft tissue swelling. Echo: no vegetations or valvular disease.

Treatment NSAIDs; corticosteroids.

Discussion Juvenile rheumatoid arthritis (JRA) most commonly affects the knee joint. Patients with JRA should undergo periodic ophthalmologic exams to carefully monitor for the onset of **iridocyclitis**, which can lead to blindness.

ID/CC	A 42-year-old woman presents with **dysphagia, butterfly rash**, arthralgias, myalgias, **skin stiffness**, swelling of the fingers, **proximal muscle weakness**, and **chronic pain in the finger joints**.
HPI	She has had these symptoms intermittently over the years, but they have worsened over the past year.
PE	VS: BP normal. PE: erythematous rash over face in butterfly distribution; **sclerodactyly**; telangiectasias in periungual areas; **nonerosive arthritis of wrist and ankle joints; proximal muscle weakness** and tenderness; weakness of neck muscles; no sensory loss; normal tendon reflexes; positive **Raynaud's phenomenon**.
Labs	Elevated ESR; **diffuse hypergammaglobulinemia; positive rheumatoid factor**; high titer of antinuclear antibodies (speckled pattern); **strongly positive test for antibody to RNP antigen** (most typical finding); anti-Smith antibody negative; anti-dsDNA antibody negative; normal complement levels; elevated **serum CPK** levels; muscle biopsy and EMG suggestive of polymyositis; **normal RFTs**.
Treatment	Corticosteroids and NSAIDs.
Discussion	Mixed connective tissue disorder (MCTD) includes characteristics of **one or more traditional connective tissue diseases at the same time**, thus making it hard to label as one or the other. These disorders include systemic lupus erythematosus, scleroderma, rheumatoid arthritis, and polymyositis.

MIXED CONNECTIVE TISSUE DISORDER

ID/CC	An **18-year-old male** presents with a **fracture of the shaft of the femur following a minor fall**.
HPI	He also complains of **facial asymmetry**, deviation of the angle of the mouth, drooling of saliva, and inability to whistle. **His father suffers from a bone disease**.
PE	Fracture of shaft of left femur; right facial nerve palsy, lower motor neuron type (entrapment neuropathy).
Labs	**Serum acid phosphatase and creatine kinase (brain isozyme) increased**; serum PTH increased; serum calcium and calcitriol normal. CBC: anemia.
Imaging	XR: **generalized symmetric osteosclerosis; "Erlenmeyer flask" deformity** of distal left femur in addition to fracture of shaft; alternating dense and lucent bands seen in metaphyses; cranium thickened and dense; paranasal and nasal sinuses underpneumatized; vertebrae show, on lateral view, **"bone in bone"** appearance.
Micro Pathology	Histopathologic studies reveal profound **deficiency of osteoclast function** and **primary spongiosa** (calcified cartilage deposited during endochondral bone formation) occurring away from growth plate (characteristic histologic finding of osteopetrosis).
Treatment	Steroid therapy with low-calcium, high-phosphate diet; management of fracture and surgical decompression of facial nerve.
Discussion	A **defect in bone resorption** secondary to **impaired osteoclast action** is the key factor in the pathogenesis of osteopetrosis.

OSTEOPETROSIS

ID/CC	A **60-year-old woman** visits her physician complaining of severe low back pain after a fall from her bed.
HPI	Onset of **menopause** was at 48 years. The patient is **not receiving hormone replacement therapy**; she suffered a Colles' fracture last year that is malunited. Directed history reveals **loss of height and a mild hunchback deformity**.
PE	Patient thin; kyphosis noted; percussion over dorsolumbar spine exquisitely tender; right wrist shows malunited Colles' fracture.
Labs	Serum calcium, phosphates, alkaline phosphatase, and PTH within normal limits; **densitometry** used to quantify osteoporosis.
Imaging	XR, dorsolumbar spine: loss of vertical height of L4 vertebra (due to collapse and compression fracture) and kyphosis. DEXA (dual-energy x-ray absorptiometry): reduced bone mass.
Gross Pathology	**Thin cortex; thin trabeculae, reduced in number**, resulting in increased medullary space; obvious fracture with healing and deformity; **collapse of vertebral bodies** with kyphoscoliosis.
Micro Pathology	Bone biopsy: thin but normally formed cortex and trabeculae; normal calcification; trabeculae very slender; microfractures and fracture healing may be evident.
Treatment	High-protein diet; **calcium and vitamin D supplementation; androgens** (anabolic effect on bone matrix); **estrogens** (shown to halt progressive bone loss); **exercise** (weight bearing acts as stimulus to bone formation); bracing of spine to prevent further fractures and deformity in a severely osteoporotic spine; bisphosphonates may be added, especially if hormone replacement therapy is contraindicated.
Discussion	Osteoporosis is characterized by a **reduction of total skeletal mass due to increased bone resorption** (bone formation is normal) with greater loss of trabecular than compact bone; it results in a predisposition to pathologic fracture. Common fracture sites are the thoracic and lumbar spine, distal forearm, and proximal femur.
Atlas Link	UCV1 PG-P3-085

RHEUMATOLOGY

ID/CC	A 44-year-old **male** with a history of hypertension develops sudden abdominal pain (due to mesenteric thrombosis) far more severe than prior episodes.
HPI	The patient had a previous episode of hematuria with peripheral edema that was diagnosed as glomerulonephritis. He has a history of intermittent fever, malaise, myalgia, arthralgia, and other vague systemic symptoms.
PE	**Livedo reticularis**; subcutaneous nodules of forearms and finger pads; painful, tympanic abdomen; purpuric spots in lower legs; **radial and peroneal nerve involvement** (MONONEURITIS MULTIPLEX).
Labs	CBC: marked neutrophilic **leukocytosis** with eosinophilia. Elevated ESR; **presence of HBsAg; positive P-ANCA**.
Imaging	Angio, renal: **multiple small aneurysms** and **infarcts**.
Gross Pathology	Fibrinoid necrotizing inflammatory infiltrate of media and adventitia of small and medium-size vessels in segmental fashion, with thrombosis and possible aneurysm formation.
Micro Pathology	Segmental areas of **fibrinoid necrosis** with neutrophilic infiltration of arterial wall.
Treatment	Steroids and other immunosuppressive agents.
Discussion	Polyarteritis nodosa is a **type III hypersensitivity reaction** characterized by **multisystem** involvement. **Renal involvement** is most common, but other presentations include pericarditis, myocardial infarction, retinal occlusion, and asthma.

ID/CC	A **70-year-old female** is seen with complaints of **inability to comb her hair, put on her coat, and get up from her chair for the past 6 months**.
HPI	She complains of **shoulder and pelvic area stiffness** and pain (especially during **morning hours**), fever, malaise, and fatigue.
PE	VS: low-grade fever. PE: pallor; stiff, deliberate movements; affected joints show restricted movement; **muscle strength normal**; remainder of physical exam normal.
Labs	CBC: **normochromic anemia. ESR markedly elevated**; other acute-phase reactants such as fibrinogen and α_2-globulin levels increased.
Imaging	XR: normal.
Treatment	Low-dose oral steroids; watch for development of giant cell arteritis, which threatens vision in up to one-third of patients.
Discussion	Polymyalgia rheumatica is characterized by **aching and morning stiffness** in the shoulder and hip girdles, the proximal extremities, the neck, and the torso; the spectrum of disease includes giant cell arteritis. Mean age at onset is 70; women are affected twice as often as men. A strong association with **HLA-DR4** has been observed. Some cases recur and some patients become steroid dependent.

POLYMYALGIA RHEUMATICA

ID/CC	A 37-year-old white female complains of **increasing weakness** for several months, especially when climbing stairs and combing her hair.
HPI	She also complains of **difficulty holding her neck upright**. For the past few weeks, she has also had **difficulty swallowing**.
PE	**Atrophy of neck, shoulder, and thigh muscles; motor weakness in all proximal muscle groups; no sensory deficit**; deep tendon reflexes reduced.
Labs	**Markedly elevated serum CPK levels; antinuclear antibodies (ANAs) demonstrable**; elevated serum transaminases and aldolase. EMG: markedly increased insertional activity; polyphasic low-amplitude motor unit action potentials with abnormally low recruitment.
Gross Pathology	Muscle edema progressing to muscle atrophy and fibrosis.
Micro Pathology	Biopsy from thigh muscles reveals **inflammatory infiltrate** in muscle, destruction of muscle fibers, and perivascular infiltrate of mononuclear cells; residual muscle fibers small.
Treatment	High-dose glucocorticoids; methotrexate; azathioprine.
Discussion	Polymyositis is frequently seen as a **paraneoplastic** manifestation of ovarian, breast, uterine, or intestinal malignancy. An associated neoplasm should always be sought.

ID/CC	A 40-year-old white female complains of **paleness and bluish discoloration of the hands, mainly upon exposure to cold, with redness upon rewarming** (RAYNAUD'S PHENOMENON); increasing pain in the knees, elbows, and hands over several months; and recent **difficulty swallowing** solid food.
HPI	She also has **masklike facies** with a limited range of expression.
PE	**Smooth, shiny, tight skin** over face and fingers; edema of hands and feet; palpable subcutaneous **calcinosis; pigmentation** and telangiectasias of face.
Labs	CBC: anemia. Hypergammaglobulinemia; anti-Scl-70 antibody; positive rheumatoid factor. PFTs: restrictive lung disease (fibrosis).
Imaging	UGI: loss of esophageal motility; dilated esophagus.
Gross Pathology	Pulmonary fibrosis with "honeycomb" appearance; swelling of esophageal wall; malabsorption syndrome; enlarged kidneys with areas of infarction; myocarditis and pericarditis.
Micro Pathology	Dense fibrosis of collagen tissue of dermis with loss of appendages and epidermal atrophy; intimal thickening of blood vessels, primarily in kidney but also in GI tract and heart.
Treatment	Supportive; calcium channel blockers; omeprazole; cisapride; penicillamine.
Discussion	Progressive systemic sclerosis (PSS) may be localized or systemic (visceral involvement) and may present with calcinosis, Raynaud's phenomenon, esophageal involvement, sclerodactyly, and telangiectasia (CREST SYNDROME).
Atlas Links	UCV1 PG-P3-089, PM-P3-089 UCV2 MC-226

RHEUMATOLOGY

PROGRESSIVE SYSTEMIC SCLEROSIS (SCLERODERMA)

ID/CC	A 60-year-old woman presents with **swelling and pain** in the left **knee after undergoing a major surgical procedure**.
HPI	She has no history of fever or trauma.
PE	Left knee warm and crepitant upon movement, which is restricted and painful; positive patellar tap indicates an effusion.
Labs	Synovial fluid from left knee shows increased leukocyte count, predominantly neutrophils; normal uric acid levels; **birefringent crystals**, both free and within leukocytes; **calcium pyrophosphate** crystals show a **weakly positive birefringence and are rhomboid in shape**.
Imaging	XR, left knee: punctate and **linear calcification in articular cartilage** (CHONDROCALCINOSIS).
Treatment	**Anti-inflammatory drugs**, including salicylates, phenylbutazone, indomethacin, and glucocorticoids, are effective to varying degrees; joint aspiration may help; triamcinolone intra-articularly for resistant cases.
Discussion	The term "pseudogout" refers to acute attacks of arthritis associated with the presence in the synovial fluid of birefringent crystals, both free and within leukocytes. **Pseudogout crystals show a weakly positive birefringence, whereas monosodium urate crystals show a strongly negative birefringence**. Generally, pseudogout crystals are also stubbier and more rhomboid than urate crystals. Radiographic evidence of calcinosis (presumably CPPD crystals) in cartilage and other structures is often present. The typical pattern involves calcification in articular cartilage, fibrocartilage (meniscus of the knee, pubic symphysis, annulus fibrosus), synovium, fibrous capsules, tendons, and bursae. Common sites of involvement include the knee, shoulder, wrist, elbow, hand, and ankle.
Atlas Link	UCV1 PM-P3-090

ID/CC	A **30-year-old** white **female** complains that the **fingers** of both hands **become pale** on **exposure to cold.**
HPI	At times, the pain is also precipitated by **emotional stress.** She is not taking any drugs and does not suffer from any other diagnosed ailment (e.g., collagen vascular disease; thyroid, adrenal, or pituitary diseases). Symptoms are relieved when she soaks her hands in warm water.
PE	Peripheral pulses palpable; **dipping patient's hands in cold water precipitated pain and resulted in development of digital blanching**; rewarming caused cyanosis and rubor of fingers.
Labs	Laboratory tests exclude all causes of secondary Raynaud's disease (collagen vascular diseases and blood dyscrasias).
Micro Pathology	Arterial wall changes in advanced state of disease.
Treatment	Protect hands and feet from exposure to cold; drug therapy with a calcium channel blocker such as nifedipine or a sympatholytic agent such as reserpine or guanethidine.
Discussion	Primary Raynaud's phenomenon, or Raynaud's disease, is a vasospastic disorder, whereas secondary Raynaud's phenomenon occurs as a complication of systemic disease such as scleroderma, systemic lupus erythematosus, and related immunologic disorders. Women are affected approximately five times more than men, and the age at presentation is usually between 30 and 40 years. The fingers are involved more frequently than the toes.

91 **RAYNAUD'S DISEASE**

ID/CC	A 23-year-old man presents with bilateral **conjunctivitis**, painful **swelling of the right knee**, bilateral heel pain, and **painless ulcers on his penis**.
HPI	He was diagnosed and treated for nongonococcal urethritis 1 week ago.
PE	Bilateral conjunctivitis with anterior uveitis; **circinate balanitis; kerato-blennorrhagicum on palms and soles**; arthritis of right knee and ankle.
Labs	**HLA-B27 positive**; synovial fluid reveals monocytes with phago-cytosed neutrophils (REITER CELLS); rheumatoid factor negative; elevated ESR.
Imaging	XR, right knee and ankle: presence of **joint effusion**.
Treatment	NSAIDs are mainstay of therapy; treat chlamydial urethritis with doxycycline.
Discussion	Reiter's syndrome is an HLA-B27-associated seronegative spondyloarthropathy that is seen almost exclusively in males and is associated with conjunctivitis, urethritis, arthritis, and heel pain. The condition has traditionally been classified as an STD, but it has also occurred following regional enteritis with *Salmonella, Shigella, Campylobacter,* and *Yersinia.*

ID/CC	A 47-year-old white **female** visits her family doctor complaining of painful swelling of the right knee.
HPI	She has a history of chronic pain along with **morning stiffness** in the hand joints **lasting** for at least **2 hours**.
PE	**Symmetrical deforming arthropathy** (ulnar deviation); soft-tissue swelling and tenderness in proximal interphalangeal and metacarpophalangeal (MCP) joint; wasting of small muscles of hand; flexion of MCP joint; hyperextension of proximal inter-phalangeal (PIP) joint and flexion of distal interphalangeal (DIP) joint (SWAN-NECK DEFORMITY); effusion on right knee with overly-ing skin redness and increased temperature; subcutaneous nodules.
Labs	Increased ESR; increased protein and white count in the synovial fluid; **positive rheumatoid factor** (IgM or IgA against IgG); positive antinuclear antibodies (ANAs); polyclonal gammopathy; associated with HLA-DR4.
Imaging	XR, plain: narrowing of joint spaces; fusion of joint (ANKYLOSIS); demineralization and bone erosions; juxta-articular osteoporosis.
Gross Pathology	Bone erosion with ankylosis; pericarditis, pleuritis; subcutaneous nodules with granuloma formation.
Micro Pathology	Plasma cell infiltration of synovial membranes (SYNOVITIS) with destruction of articular cartilage, tendons, and ligaments by thickened, **inflamed synovial tissue** (PANNUS); **fibrosis**.
Treatment	Physical therapy, thermal compresses, splints; NSAIDs; methotrexate; gold; chloroquine; corticosteroids; other immunosuppressants; surgery.
Discussion	Rheumatoid arthritis is the most **common autoimmune disease**. Ocular involvement is seen in 5% of cases; neurologic involve-ment of the carpal tunnel can be a complication.
Atlas Link	UCV2 IM2-055

RHEUMATOLOGY

ID/CC	A 47-year-old woman visits her health care center complaining of **dryness of the mouth** (XEROSTOMIA) and a **gritty sensation in her eyes with dryness** (XEROPHTHALMIA).
HPI	She has been hypertensive for 20 years and has suffered from long-standing **rheumatoid arthritis**, for which she has been treated with NSAIDs.
PE	**Filamentous keratitis with areas of denuded corneal epithelium** (KERATOCONJUNCTIVITIS SICCA) on slit-lamp examination with rose bengal dye staining of cornea; **diminished tear formation** as measured on strip of filter paper, with one end of paper placed inside lower eyelid (SCHIRMER TEST); **parotid enlargement**; excessively dry mouth with abundant dental caries; characteristic swan-neck deformities of hands and ulnar deviation (due to long-standing deforming rheumatoid arthritis).
Labs	Low saliva flow rates with lemon juice stimulation (< 0.5 mL/ min); hypergammaglobulinemia; **positive antibodies to IgG globulins** (RHEUMATOID FACTOR) and **antinuclear antibodies (ANAs)**.
Imaging	Sialography (x-rays following cannulation and contrast injection of parotid ducts): distortion of normal arborization pattern. Nuc: impaired salivary function.
Micro Pathology	Salivary and lacrimal glands show inflammatory infiltration with T cells, B cells, and plasma cells, with predominance of CD4+ T cells; **ductal obstruction** with glandular acinar tissue atrophy with fatty change.
Treatment	Artificial tear preparations, increased and frequent oral intake of fluids, careful dental hygiene, plaque control programs, fluoride application.
Discussion	Sjögren's syndrome is defined as autoimmune destruction of salivary and lacrimal glands; it may be primary or associated with other autoimmune diseases.

ID/CC	An 18-year-old white **female** presents with a **malar rash** that is exacerbated by sun exposure (PHOTOSENSITIVITY) as well as with arthralgias and **joint stiffness** involving her ankles, wrists, and knee joints; she also complains of decreased visual acuity, anorexia, weight loss, malaise, and weakness.
HPI	She has a history of hematuria and no history of drug intake prior to the onset of symptoms.
PE	VS: hypertension (BP 160/100). PE: pallor; malar rash; painful restriction of movement of wrist, knee, and ankle joints; no obvious deformity; whitish exudates in cytoid bodies on funduscopic exam.
Labs	CBC: Coombs-positive **anemia; neutropenia; thrombocytopenia. Decreased C1q, C2, C4; positive antinuclear antibodies (ANAs), anti-native DNA, and anti-Sm antibodies**; positive LE cells; false-positive VDRL due to antiphospholipid antibodies. UA: protein-uria; RBCs and **RBC casts**.
Imaging	XR, plain: no erosive changes. Echo: no vegetations seen on valves (vs. endocarditis).
Gross Pathology	Serositis; pericarditis; pleuritis; splenomegaly; hyperkeratotic, erythematous plaques.
Micro Pathology	Thickening of basement membrane on renal biopsy; mesangial proliferation; thickened capillary walls, creating **"wire-loop"** appearance; diffuse proliferative glomerulonephritis; immune complex deposition in skin with lymphocytic infiltration; vasculitis with fibrinoid necrosis of small arteries; almost any organ may be involved.
Treatment	High-dose corticosteroids for prolonged periods; alternative drugs: chloroquine; cyclophosphamide as treatment for lupus nephritis.
Discussion	Systemic lupus erythematosus (SLE) is a **type III hypersensitivity reaction**. Immune complex vasculitis is the basic pathologic lesion; can be drug-induced (e.g., hydralazine, procainamide, isoniazid).
Atlas Links	UCV1 **PM-P3-095** UCV2 IM2-056

RHEUMATOLOGY

SYSTEMIC LUPUS ERYTHEMATOSUS (SLE)

ID/CC A 45-year-old **white** male complains of chronic nasal congestion and discharge over the past 5 months.

HPI Ten days ago he developed an earache and cough along with bloody sputum production, dyspnea, muscle pain, red eyes, fever, and night sweats.

PE Dried-up crusts of mucus in congestive nasal mucosa with shallow **ulcers and perforation of the nasal septum**; sibilant rales disseminated in lung fields.

Labs CBC: mild anemia; moderate leukocytosis. UA: numerous RBCs; **red cell casts** and granular casts in urine. **Positive cytoplasmic antineutrophilic antibodies (C-ANCA)** in serum.

Imaging CXR: bilateral scattered small nodular densities with no hilar adenopathy (vs. sarcoid).

Gross Pathology Granuloma formation in lungs; vasculitis and inflammation involving **upper respiratory tract**, lungs, peripheral arteries, and **kidneys**.

Micro Pathology Focal necrotizing vasculitis involving small vessels; granulomas and crescentic glomerulonephritis.

Treatment Immunosuppressive therapy with steroids and cyclophosphamide.

Discussion Wegener's granulomatosis is a systemic **autoimmune vasculitis** that consists of necrotizing vasculitis and necrotizing granulomas of the lungs and airways, as well as a necrotizing glomerulitis. C-ANCA is seen in the majority of patients and serves as a marker of disease activity.

Atlas Link UCV1 PM-P3-096

ID/CC   A 58-year-old male complains of **headache**, anxiety, shortness of breath, and increased sleepiness (SOMNOLENCE) while experiencing an **acute exacerbation of COPD**.

HPI   The patient is a **chronic smoker** and also complains of recent **blurring of vision**. He has a history of episodic shortness of breath, mucoid cough, and occasional wheezing (consistent with predominantly **bronchitic COPD**) but no history of neurologic deficit, previous hypertension, or diabetes.

PE   VS: tachycardia; tachypnea; mild systolic hypertension; no fever. PE: anxious and in moderate respiratory distress; using accessory muscles of respiration with prolonged expiration; mild **central cyanosis and pallor; no clubbing**; extremities warm; **flapping tremor of hand** (ASTERIXIS); **bounding pulses** (due to high volume); funduscopy reveals **early papilledema**; chest barrel-shaped with bilateral rhonchi and occasional rales; no focal neurologic deficits.

Labs   ABGs: **hypoxia, hypercapnia, and partially compensated respiratory acidosis**. CBC: polycythemia.

Imaging   CXR (PA view): increased bronchovascular markings (dirty lung fields).

Treatment   **Low-dose continuous oxygen inhalation and, if required, mechanical ventilation** to reverse acidosis; broad-spectrum antibiotics, bronchodilators (ipratropium bromide and sympathomimetics), and steroids are used in COPD patients.

Discussion   Dyspnea and headache are the cardinal symptoms of hypercapnia. Hypercapnia also produces a variety of neurologic abnormalities; symptoms include somnolence, blurred vision, restlessness, and anxiety that can progress to tremors, asterixis, delirium, and coma. Supplemental oxygen should be used sparingly to avoid increasing PaO_2, which removes the hypoxic respiratory stimulus and leads to respiratory depression.

TOXICOLOGY